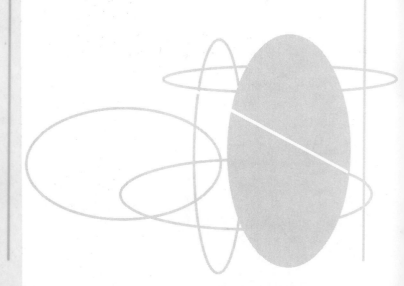

DORLAND'S
HEMATOLOGY/ ONCOLOGY SPELLER

Consultant

GEORGE P. CANELLOS, MD
William Rosenberg Professor of Medicine,
Harvard Medical School;
Chief, Division of Medical Oncology,
Dana-Farber Cancer Institute;
Physician, Brigham and Women's Hospital,
Boston, Massachusetts

Consultant for Syllabication

CAROL A. HART, PhD
Narberth, Pennsylvania

DORLAND'S
HEMATOLOGY/ ONCOLOGY SPELLER

W.B. SAUNDERS COMPANY
A Division of Harcourt Brace & Company
Philadelphia London Toronto Montreal Sydney Tokyo

W.B. SAUNDERS COMPANY
A Division of
Harcourt Brace & Company

The Curtis Center
Independence Square West
Philadelphia, Pennsylvania 19106

Library of Congress Cataloging-in-Publication Data

Dorland's hematology/oncology speller.

    p.   cm.

ISBN 0–7216–3750–7

    1. Oncology—Terminology.   2. Hematology—
    Terminology.   I. W.B. Saunders Company.
    II. Title: Hematology/oncology speller.
    [DNLM: 1. Medical Oncology—nomenclature.
    2. Hematology—nomenclature. WH 15 D711]

RC 254.5.D64   1993

616.1′5′0014—dc20

DNLM/DLC   92–13352

DORLAND'S HEMATOLOGY/   ISBN 0–7216–3750–7
ONCOLOGY SPELLER

Printed in the United States of America.

Last digit is the print number: 9   8   7   6   5   4   3   2

Preface

The specialties of hematology and oncology are characterized by rapid advances and an accompanying explosion of terminology. The purpose of *Dorland's Hematology/Oncology Speller* is to present a comprehensive listing of terms used in these specialties, together with a system of acceptable end-of-line breaks. In order to make the book easier to use, multiple listings have been given for hard to find terms, such as eponyms, which will be found not only at the thing named but also at each proper name in the term.

The word list has been compiled from a variety of sources, including the *Dorland's Illustrated Medical Dictionary* database and a number of texts, monographs, and journals. Chemotherapy regimens have been given great emphasis in the word list. A large number of terms from immunohematology have also been included. Two useful appendices organize the antigenic determinants, genotypes, and phenotypes of blood group systems and the specificities of HLA antigens.

Special thanks are owed to our consultant, George P. Canellos, MD, who reviewed the list of terms, and also to Carol A. Hart, PhD, our consultant for hyphenation, for their valued and valuable work in the preparation of this book.

DOUGLAS M. ANDERSON
Chief Lexicographer

How This Book Is Arranged

Order of Entries

Dorland's Hematology/Oncology Speller follows the same scheme of arrangement as *Dorland's Illustrated Medical Dictionary*. Main entries follow one another in letter-by-letter alphabetical order regardless of spaces or hyphens that occur within them (see below for special rules for chemical names); compound entries consisting of one or more adjectives and a noun will be found as subentries under the noun. In some cases where there might be a question about where to look to find an entry, entries have been given in more than one place, even under an adjective.

Eponymic terms. Terms containing a proper name are given multiple listings, once under the thing named and once under each eponym. Thus the following entries appear for *Reed-Sternberg cells:*

cell
  Reed-Sternberg c's

Reed
  R.-Sternberg cells

Sternberg
  Reed-S. cells

Umlauts are ignored for alphabetization, and proper names beginning *Mc* or *Mac* are alphabetized as though spelled *Mac*.

Chemical prefixes. Italicized chemical prefixes such as the letters *p*- and *o*- and *cis*- and *trans*-, together with numbers, Greek letters, and the small capitals L- and D-, do not count for alphabetization. When prefixes are written out in full, however, as *para-* instead of *p*-, they are counted for alphabetical order.

Subentries

Each subentry appears on a new line following the main entry and is indented. The main entry word in a subentry is represented only by the initial letter, as *B cell l.* under *lymphoma*, with three exceptions. For regular English plurals, the abbreviation is the initial letter followed by *'s* (as *l's* for *lymphomas*). For irregular or Greek or Latin plurals, the entire plural form is written out in full.

For possessive forms, the initial letter is followed by *'s* (as *F's anemia* for *Fanconi's anemia*). In subentries the main entry word is ignored for alphabetization, as are prepositions, conjunctions, and articles.

Possessive Forms

The use of the possessive in eponyms is controversial. This book follows the example of *Dorland's Illustrated Medical Dictionary,* that is, the *'s* is favored where the sources for a term justify its appearance. Whether or not to use the possessive form is a matter left to the individual; owing to the present lack of consistency and consensus, no prescription can be given. There are of course some terms in which the possessive is never used, as *Christmas disease.*

Abbreviations and Acronyms

A number of abbreviations and acronyms are given, together with the words or phrases that they stand for. The selection is of course only a small fraction of the abbreviations and acronyms in actual use. If more than one word or phrase is listed with an abbreviation, the terms are given in alphabetical order and each additional term is placed on a new line and indented.

Word Divisions

Acceptable word divisions are given for main entries; syllabication is based on pronunciation. Not all syllable breaks are shown; for example, because single letters at the beginnings and ends of words may not be separated from the rest of the word, such divisions are not given. Likewise, single letters should not be separated from the word elements they belong to in compound words. Breaks that could confuse the reader as to the meaning of a word are to be avoided. In many cases, words may be broken at places other than the ones that appear in this book (for example, different pronunciations imply different word breaks); it is impossible to show every break that could occur for every word. What appears here is one possible system.

Alternative Spellings

A number of words have alternative spellings, ranging from the difference of a single letter to the use of variant forms of Greek and Latin stems. Although every effort has been made to ensure that the spellings included in this book are valid, no indications of preference are given.

Brackets and Parentheses

Some entries require a bit of explanation; these explanations are enclosed in parentheses. Brackets are sometimes used as a part of Latin anatomical nomenclature to enclose an eponym in the genitive case; in this book such eponyms generally appear all lower case (as in *Dorland's Illustrated Medical Dictionary*), but an initial capital for the name is acceptable.

Plurals

Plurals for foreign words, nearly all of them Greek and Latin, are given with the appropriate entries. In addition, they are given again as separate entries if they do not occur within a few lines of the singular form.

Contents

AACR
American Association for
Cancer Research

AAFC
flurocitabine

Aase
A. syndrome

Ab·bé
A.-Zeiss apparatus
A.-Zeiss counting cell
A.-Zeiss counting chamber

Ab·bott
A.-Parker LifeCare 1500
Ambulatory Microinfusor
A.-Parker LifeCare 1500
pump

ABCD
doxorubicin, bleomycin, lomustine, and dacarbazine
doxorubicin, bleomycin, lomustine, and dexametha-
sone

ABDIC
doxorubicin, bleomycin
sulfate, dacarbazine, lo-
mustine, and prednisone

ABDV
doxorubicin, bleomycin
sulfate, dacarbazine, and
vinblastine

Abel·son
A. murine leukemia virus

Ab·er·ne·thy
A's sarcoma

ab·er·ra·tion
chromosome a.

Abi·plat·in

Abi·trate

ab·la·tion
adrenal a.
ovarian a.

abl gene

abl on·co·gene

ABMT
allogeneic bone marrow
transplantation
autologous bone marrow
transplantation

ab·nor·mal·i·ty
B-cell a.
chromosomal a.
chromosome a.
clonal a.
Dynia a.
gene a.
genetic a.
immunologic a.
karyotype a.
karyotypic a.
leukemic cell a's
metabolic a.
platelet a's
T-cell a.

ABOS
doxorubicin, bleomycin
sulfate, vincristine, and
streptozotocin

ABP
doxorubicin, bleomycin,
prednisone

Abri·ko·sov (Abri·kos·soff)
A's tumor

ab·scess
splenic a.

ab·sorp·ti·om·e·try
single-photon a.

1

ABVD
> doxorubicin, bleomycin, vinblastine, and dacarbazine

ABVP
> doxorubicin, bleomycin sulfate, teniposide, and prednisone
> doxorubicin, bleomycin sulfate, vinblastine, and prednisone
> doxorubicin, bleomycin sulfate, vincristine, and prednisone

AC
> doxorubicin and cyclophosphamide

acan·tho·cyte

acan·tho·cy·to·sis

ac·an·tho·ma *pl.* ac·an·tho·mas, ac·an·tho·ma·ta

acan·thro·cyte

acan·thro·cy·to·sis

ac·cel·er·a·tor
> a. globulin
> linear a.
> serum prothrombin conversion a. (SPCA)
> serum thrombotic a.

ac·cel·er·in

ac·cess
> vascular a.

Ac·cus·pin

Ac·cu·trol

ACD (acid citrate dextrose) whole blood

ac·e·tab·u·lum *pl.* ac·e·tab·u·li

ac·et·a·zol·a·mide

ac·e·tyl·cho·lin·es·ter·ase

ac·e·tyl·cys·te·ine

N-ac·e·tyl-L-ly·sine meth·yl es·ter

AcG
> accelerator globulin (coagulation factor V)

ac·id
> aminocaproic a.
> ε-aminocaproic a.
> η-aminocaproic a.
> aminolevulinic a.
> arachidonic a.
> 13-azaprostanoic a.
> bile a's
> citric a.
> deoxy-manno-octulosonic a.
> deoxyribonucleic a. (DNA)
> epsilon-aminocaproic a.
> ethacrynic a.
> fatty a.
> a. ferrocyanide
> flavone acetic a.
> folic a.
> hydrochloric a.
> 12-hydroxyeicosatetraenoic a.
> 12-hydroxyheptadecatrienoic a.
> 13-hydroxyoctadecadienoic a.
> hypochlorous a.
> hypothiocyanous a.
> keto-deoxyoctonic a.
> linoleic a.
> methylmalonic a.
> nalidixic a.
> octonic a.
> phenolphthalein glucuronic a.
> phosphatidic a.
> phosphotungstic a.
> *cis*-retinoic a.
> *trans*-retinoic a.
> tranexamic a.
> trichloroacetic a.

ac·id *(continued)*
    trimethylcolchicinic a.
    trinitrobenzene sulfonic a.
    uric a.
    vanillylmandelic a.

ac·i·de·mia
    methylmalonic a.

acid·o·cyte

ac·i·do·sis
    lactic a.
    metabolic a.
    respiratory a.

ac·id phos·pha·tase

ac·id·uria
    amino a.
    orotic a.

Aci·ne·to·bac·ter
    A. calcoaceticus

ac·i·vi·cin

acla·cin·o·my·cin

ACNU
    nimustine

Acnu
    nimustine

A-COMLA

ACP
    acid phosphatase

AcP
    acid phosphatase

ac·ral

ac·ri·din·yl an·is·i·dide

acro·le·in

ac·ry·lo·ni·trile

ACST
    autologous stem cell trans-
        plantation

ACTH
    adrenocorticotropic hor-
        mone

ACTH 4,9 [ACTH (4-9)]

Ac·thar

Ac·ti·dil

ac·tin

ac·ti·no·my·cin

ac·ti·no·my·cin D

ac·ti·va·tion
    complement a.
    contact a.
    factor a.
    lymphocyte a.
    metabolic a.
    neutrophil a.
    platelet a.
    protein kinase a.

ac·ti·va·tor
    plasminogen a.
    polyclonal a.
    prothrombin a.
    tissue-type plasminogen a.
    two-chain urokinase-type
        plasminogen a.
    urokinase-type plasmino-
        gen a. (u-PA)

ac·ti·vin A

ac·tiv·i·ty
    antineoplastic a.
    antitumor a.
    B cell–derived burst pro-
        moting a. (B-BPA)
    burst-promoting a. (BPA)
    colony-inhibiting a.
    colony-stimulating a.
    a's of daily living
    graft vs leukemia a.
    leukemia-associated inhib-
        itory a. (LIA)
    leukemia cell–derived in-
        hibitory a.
    leukocyte procoagulant a.

ac·tiv·i·ty *(continued)*
    mitotic a.
    natural suppressor a.

acu·men·tin

acu·punc·ture

Acu·stain

Acu·tase

acy·clo·vir
    a. sodium

ac·yl·trans·fer·ase
    phospholipid a's
    pituitary a.

ADCB
    doxorubicin, dacarbazine,
        lomustine, and bleomycin
        sulfate

ADCC
    antibody-dependent cell-
        mediated cytotoxicity

ad·duct
    hemoglobin/spectrin a.
    platinum-DNA a.

ad·e·nine
    a. nucleotide

ad·e·no·ac·an·tho·ma

ad·e·no·can·croid

ad·e·no·car·ci·no·ma
    acinar a.
    acinous a.
    alveolar a.
    a. of breast
    a. of cervix
    clear cell a.
    a. of colon
    a. of endometrium
    a. of esophagus
    a. of exocrine pancreas
    follicular a.
    a. of gallbladder
    invasive a.
    a. of kidney

ad·e·no·car·ci·no·ma *(continued)*
    a. of lung
    a. of mediastinum
    mucinous a.
    mucin-producing a.
    papillary a.
    polypoid a.
    a. of small intestine
    a. of stomach
    a. of thyroid gland
    a. of uterus
    a. of vagina

ad·e·no·cele

ad·e·no·chon·dro·ma

ad·e·no·cyst

ad·e·no·cys·to·ma
    papillary a. lymphomato-
        sum

ad·e·no·ep·i·the·li·o·ma

ad·e·no·fi·bro·ma
    a. edematodes

ad·e·no·leio·myo·fi·bro·ma

ad·e·no·li·po·ma

ad·e·no·li·po·ma·to·sis

ad·e·no·lym·pho·ma

ad·e·no·ma
    acidophilic a.
    adrenal a.
    a. of adrenal cortex
    adrenal cortical a.
    a. alveolare
    basal cell a.
    basophil a.
    basophilic a.
    bronchial a's
    carcinoid a. of bronchus
    chief cell a.
    chromophobe a.
    chromophobic a.
    clear cell a.
    cortical a's
    eosinophil a.

ad·e·no·ma *(continued)*
   a. fibrosum
   follicular a.
   a. gelatinosum
   a. hidradenoides
   Hürthle cell a.
   hyperfunctioning adrenal
    cortical a.
   islet a.
   a's of kidney
   langerhansian a.
   malignant a.
   monomorphic a.
   mucinous a.
   multiple a's
   nephrogenic a.
   a. ovarii testiculare
   oxyphilic granular cell a.
   papillary cystic a.
   a. of parathyroid glands
   pituitary a.
   pleomorphic a.
   racemose a.
   a. of salivary glands
   sebaceous a.
   a. sebaceum
   serrated a.
   a. sudoriparum
   tubular a.
   a. tubulare testiculare
    ovarii
   tubulovillous a.
   villous a.

ad·e·no·ma·toid

ad·e·no·ma·to·sis
   multiple endocrine a.
   pluriglandular a.
   polyendocrine a.
   pulmonary a.

ad·e·no·ma·tous

ad·e·no·myo·ep·i·the·li·o·
ma

ad·e·no·myo·fi·bro·ma

ad·e·no·my·o·ma
   a. psammopapillare

ad·e·no·my·o·ma·to·sis

ad·e·no·my·o·ma·tous

ad·e·no·myo·sar·co·ma
   embryonal a.

ad·e·nop·a·thy
   axillary a.
   cervical a.
   malignant a.
   thoracic a.

ad·e·no·sar·co·ma
   embryonal a.

aden·o·sine
   a. diphosphate (ADP)
   a. triphosphate (ATP)

aden·o·sine de·am·i·nase

ad·e·no·sis

ad·e·no·squa·mous

aden·yl·ate

aden·yl·ate syn·the·tase

ADH
   antidiuretic hormone

ad·her·ence
   immune a.

ad·her·ent

ad·he·sin

ad·he·sion
   abdominal a.
   cell a.
   platelet a.
   postoperative a.

ad·he·sive·ness
   platelet a.

ADIC
   doxorubicin and dacarbazine

ad·i·po·cyte

ad·i·po·fi·bro·ma

ad·ju·vant
    A. 65
    Freund's a.

ad·ju·van·tic·i·ty

ADOC
    cisplatin, doxorubicin, vin-
        cristine, and cyclophos-
        phamide

ADP
    adenosine diphosphate

ADR
    doxorubicin (Adriamycin)

Adr
    doxorubicin (Adriamycin)

ad·re·nal

adren·a·lin·emia

adre·no·cor·ti·cal

adre·no·cor·ti·coid
    glucocorticoid a's

Adri·a·my·cin

Adri·a·my·cin PFS

Adri·a·my·cin RDF

Adru·cil

ad·sorp·tion
    agglutinin a.
    immune a.

AF
    accelerated fractionation

af·fin·i·ty
    a. crosslinking

afi·brin·o·gen·emia
    congenital a.
    hereditary a.

af·la·tox·in

AFP
    alpha-fetoprotein

af·ter·load·ing

AFX
    accelerated fractionation

agam·ma·glob·u·lin·emia
    Bruton's a.
    common variable a.
    lymphopenic a.
    Swiss type a.
    X-linked a.
    X-linked infantile a.

agen·cy
    International A. for Re-
        search on Cancer

agent
    alkylating a.
    analgesic a.
    antiemetic a.
    antimicrotubule a.
    antineoplastic a.
    antiparasitic a.
    antiplatelet a.
    antisickling a.
    antiviral a.
    carcinogenic a.
    cardioprotective a.
    chemotherapeutic a.
    chemotherapy a.
    contrast a.
    cytotoxic a.
    delta a.
    paramagnetic contrast a.
    sclerosing a.

ag·glu·ti·na·tion
    cold a.
    cross a.
    intravascular a.
    passive a.
    platelet a.
    ristocetin-induced platelet
        a. (RIPA)

ag·glu·ti·na·tor

ag·glu·ti·nin
    anti-Rh a.
    chief a.
    cold a.
    complete a.

ag·glu·ti·nin *(continued)*
    cross a.
    cross-reacting a.
    group a.
    immune a.
    incomplete a.
    leukocyte a.
    major a.
    minor a.
    partial a.
    platelet a.
    saline a.
    T a.
    warm a.

ag·glu·tin·o·gen

ag·glu·ti·no·gen·ic

ag·glu·ti·no·phil·ic

ag·glu·to·gen·ic

ag·gre·ga·tion
    platelet a.
    ristocetin-induced platelet
        a. (RIPA)

ag·gre·gin

ag·gre·gom·e·ter

ag·gre·gom·e·try

ag·gres·sive

ag·gres·sive·ness

agly·ce·mia

ag·o·nist

agran·u·lo·cyte

agran·u·lo·cy·to·sis
    drug-induced a.
    infantile genetic a.

ahap·to·glo·bin·emia

AHF
    accelerated hyperfraction-
        ation

AHG
    antihemophilic globulin

A-hydro·Cort

AIDS
    acquired immune defi-
        ciency syndrome
    acquired immunodefi-
        ciency syndrome

AILD
    angioimmunoblastic
        lymphadenopathy with
        dysproteinemia

AISA
    acquired idiopathic sidero-
        blastic anemia

AJCC
    American Joint Commit-
        tee on Cancer

AJCC/UICC staging (for
    colorectal carcinoma)

al·a·no·sine

Alax·in

al·bu·min
    a. A
    blood a.
    iodinated I 131 a.
    serum a.

al·bu·min·emia

al·bu·min·uria
    Bamberger's hematogenic
        a.

al·co·hol
    denatured a.

Al·der
    A.'s constitutional granu-
        lation anomaly
    A.-Reilly anomaly

al·des·leu·kin

al·do·lase

al·do·lase de·fi·cien·cy

al·do·ster·on·ism
    primary a.

al·do·ster·o·no·ma

Al·drich
    A's syndrome
    Wiskott-A. syndrome

aleu·ke·mia

aleu·ke·mic

aleu·kia
    a. hemorrhagica

aleu·ko·cyt·ic

aleu·ko·cy·to·sis

al·fa·cal·ci·dol

Al·fer·on N

ALK
    melphalan (Alkeran)

al·ka·le·mia

al·ka·line phos·pha·tase
    placental a.p.

al·ka·loid
    vinca a's

Al·ker·an

al·kyl·at·ing

ALL
    acute lymphoblastic leuke-
        mia

al·lele

Al·ler·act

al·lo·an·ti·body

al·lo·an·ti·gen
    allo-BMT allogeneic bone
        transplantation

al·lo·ep·i·tope

al·lo·ge·ne·ic

al·lo·gen·ic

al·lo·im·mune

al·lo·im·mu·ni·za·tion

al·lo·pur·i·nol

al·lo·trans·plant

al·lot·ri·odon·tia

al·lo·type
    Am a's
    Gm a's
    Inv a's
    Km a's
    Oz a.

al·lo·typ·ic

al·lo·ty·py

Al·ma·cone

Al·ma·cone II

al·o·pe·cia
    chemotherapy-induced a.

ALP
    alkaline phosphatase

al·pha-L-id·uron·i·dase

al·pha-L-id·uron·i·dase de·fi·
    cien·cy

al·pha·nine

al·pha$_2$ PI
    alpha$_2$-plasmin inhibitor

al·pha-spec·trin

al·pha-to·coph·er·ol

al·pra·zo·lam

al·ter·ation
    chromosomal a's

al·tret·amine

Alu·drox

alu·mi·na
    a. and magnesia
    a. and magnesium carbon-
        ate
    a. and magnesium trisili-
        cate
    a., magnesia, and calcium
        carbonate

alu·mi·na *(continued)*
  a., magnesia, and simethi-
    cone
  magnesium trisilicate, a.,
    and magnesia
  a., magnesium trisilicate,
    and sodium bicarbonate
  simethicone, a., calcium
    carbonate, and magnesia
  simethicone, a., magne-
    sium carbonate, and
    magnesia

alu·mi·num
  basic a. carbonate
  a. hydroxide

al·ve·o·lus *pl.* al·ve·o·li

alym·pho·cy·to·sis

alym·pho·pla·sia
  thymic a.

α_2 M
  α_2 macroglobulin

am·bo·cep·tor

amelo·blas·to·ma
  melanotic a.
  pigmented a.
  pituitary a.

Amen

Amer·i·can As·so·ci·a·tion
  for Can·cer Re·search

Amer·i·can Can·cer So·ci·e·
  ty

Amer·i·can Joint Com·mit·
  tee on Can·cer

Amer·i·can Joint Com·mit·
  tee on Can·cer clas·si·fi·ca·
  tion (for extraocular
  melanoma)

Amer·i·can Joint Com·mit·
  tee on Can·cer Per·form·
  ance Sta·tus Scale

Amer·i·can Joint Com·mit·
  tee for Can·cer Stag·ing
  and End Re·sults Re·port·
  ing

Amer·i·can My·co·sis Fun·
  goid·es Co·op·er·a·tive
  Group sys·tem (for staging
  of mycosis fungoides)

Amer·i·can So·ci·ety of Clin·
  i·cal On·col·o·gy

Amer·i·can So·ci·ety for
  Ther·a·peu·tic Ra·di·ol·o·
  gy

Ames
  A. test

A-metha·Pred

ameth·op·ter·in

Am·i·car

ami·fos·tine

amil·o·ride
  a. and hydrochlorothiazide

amine

ami·no·ac·id·emia

o-ami·no·azo·tol·u·ene

4-ami·no·bi·phen·yl

ami·no·ca·pro·ic acid

ε-ami·no·ca·pro·ic acid

η-ami·no·ca·pro·ic acid

ami·no·glu·teth·i·mide

ami·no·gly·co·side

8-ami·no·guan·o·sine

ami·no·lev·u·lin·ic acid

am·i·nop·ter·in

2-ami·no·pu·rine

ami·no·thi·a·da·zole

am·i·trip·ty·line

AML-193 leukemic cell line

AML-WC (myelomonocytic)
   cell line

am·mo·ni·um
   potassium gluconate, po-
     tassium citrate, and a.
     chloride

am·o·na·fide

AMP
   adenosine monophosphate

am·phi·car·ci·no·gen·ic

am·phi·crine

am·phi·leu·ke·mic

Am·pho·jel Plus

am·pho·phil·ic

am·pho·ter·i·cin

am·pli·fi·ca·tion
   gene a.
   N-*myc* a.

ampulla *pl.* am·pul·lae
   a. of Vater

am·pu·ta·tion

AMSA
   amsacrine

Amsa
   amsacrine

am·sa·crine

am·y·lase

am·yl·emia

am·y·loid

am·y·loi·do·sis
   immunocyte-derived a.
   immunocytic a.
   senile a.
   systemic a.

An·a·bol·in LA-100

an·ac·me·sis

an·a·gre·lide

an·ak·me·sis

an·al·bu·min·emia

an·al·ge·sia

an·al·ge·sic
   opioid a.

an·a·logue
   adenosine a.
   purine a.
   somatostatin a.

anal·y·sis *pl.* anal·y·ses
   cytochemical a.
   flow cytometric a.
   genetic probe a.
   heteroduplex a.
   karyotype a.
   karyotypic a.
   limiting dilution a.
   linkage a.
   morphometric a.
   Northern a.
   Northern blot a.
   Southern a.
   Southern blot a.
   steroid hormone receptor
     a.
   Western blot a.

an·an·a·phy·lax·is

ana·phy·lac·tic

ana·phy·lac·to·gen

ana·phy·lac·to·gen·e·sis

ana·phy·lac·to·gen·ic

ana·phy·lac·toid

ana·phy·la·tox·in

ana·phy·lax·is
   active a.
   aggregate a.
   antiserum a.
   generalized a.
   inverse a.
   passive a.

ana·phy·lax·is *(continued)*
   reverse a.
   systemic a.

an·a·pla·sia
   monophasic a.
   polyphasic a.

an·a·plas·tia

an·a·plas·tic

an·as·to·mo·sis *pl.* an·as·to·mo·ses
   coloanal a.
   ileocolic a.
   ileorectal a.

Ana·var

an·crod

an·drei·o·ma

an·dreo·blas·to·ma

An·dro 100

An·dro·cur

An·dro-Cyp

an·dro·gen
   antitumor a.

an·dro·gen·ic

An·droid

An·dro L.A. 200

An·dro·lone

An·dro·lone-50

An·dro·lone D

an·dro·ma

An·dro·naq-50

An·dro·naq-LA

An·dro·nate

An·dro·pos·i·to·ry 100

An·dryl 200

ane·mia
   achrestic a.
   achylic a.
   a. achylica
   acquired idiopathic sidero-blastic a.
   acquired infectious hemo-lytic a.
   acquired sideroachrestic a.
   acute a.
   acute acquired hemolytic a.
   acute posthemorrhagic a.
   Addison's a.
   Addison-Biermer a.
   addisonian a.
   aplastic a.
   aregenerative a.
   aregenerative a., chronic congenital
   autoimmune hemolytic a. (AIHA)
   Bartonella a.
   Blackfan-Diamond a.
   cameloid a.
   cardiac hemolytic a.
   chronic disorder a.
   a. of chronic disorders
   chronic hemolytic a. with paroxysmal nocturnal hemoglobinuria
   chronic hypochromic a.
   chronic nonspherocytic he-molytic a.
   chronic refractory a. with sideroblastic bone mar-row
   cold antibody autoimmune hemolytic a.
   congenital aregenerative a.
   congenital dyserythropoi-etic a.
   congenital Heinz body he-molytic a.
   congenital hemolytic a.
   congenital hypoplastic a.
   congenital a. of newborn

ane·mia *(continued)*

    congenital nonspherocytic a.

    congenital nonspherocytic hemolytic a.

    congenital pernicious a.

    congenital sideroachrestic a.

    constitutional aplastic a.

    Cooley's a.

    copper deficiency a.

    Diamond-Blackfan a.

    dilution a.

    dilutional a.

    dimorphic a.

    drug-induced Coombs-positive hemolytic a.

    drug-induced hemolytic a.

    drug-induced immune hemolytic a.

    elliptocytary a.

    elliptocytic hemolytic a.

    elliptocytotic a.

    erythroblastic a. of childhood

    essential a.

    familial erythroblastic a.

    familial hypoplastic a.

    familial splenic a.

    Fanconi's a.

    fetal a.

    folic acid deficiency a.

    glucose-6-phosphate dehydrogenase deficiency a.

    glucose-6-phosphate dehydrogenase deficiency hemolytic a.

    Heinz-body a's

    hemolytic a.

    hemolytic a., acquired

    hemolytic a., acute

    hemolytic a., congenital

    hemolytic a., congenital nonspherocytic

    hemolytic a., hereditary nonspherocytic

    hemolytic a., immune

    hemolytic a., infectious

ane·mia *(continued)*

    hemolytic a., microangiopathic

    hemolytic a., toxic

    hemorrhagic a.

    hereditary hemolytic a.

    hereditary iron-loading a.

    hereditary nonspherocytic a.

    hereditary primary sideroblastic a.

    hereditary sideroachrestic a.

    hereditary sideroblastic a.

    hereditary spherocytic hemolytic a.

    hypochromic a.

    hypochromic a., idiopathic

    hypochromic microcytic a.

    a. hypochromica siderochrestica hereditaria

    hypoplastic a.

    hypoplastic a., congenital

    hypoplastic congenital a.

    hypoplastic congenital a. of Blackfan and Diamond

    hypoproliferative a.

    idiopathic a.

    idiopathic acquired sideroblastic a.

    idiopathic autoimmune hemolytic a.

    idiopathic refractory sideroblastic a.

    immune hemolytic a.

    immunohemolytic a.

    infectious hemolytic a.

    iron deficiency a.

    iron-loading a.

    juvenile pernicious a.

    leukoerythroblastic a.

    macrocytic a.

    macrocytic a., nutritional

    macrocytic megaloblastic a.

    Mediterranean a.

    megaloblastic a.

    megaloblastic a., familial

ane·mia *(continued)*
  megaloblastic a. of infancy
  megalocytic a.
  microangiopathic a.
  microcytic a.
  milk a.
  myelopathic a.
  myelophthisic a.
  a. neonatorum
  nonfamilial splenic a.
  nonspherocytic hemolytic a.
  normochromic a.
  normocytic a.
  nutritional macrocytic a.
  osteosclerotic a.
  paraneoplastic a.
  pernicious a.
  pernicious a., juvenile
  physiologic a.
  physiologic a. of infancy
  polar a.
  posthemorrhagic a.
  posthemorrhagic a., acute
  posthemorrhagic a. of newborn
  postsurgical macrocytic a.
  primaquine-sensitive a.
  primary a.
  primary acquired sideroblastic a.
  pure red cell a.
  pyridoxine-responsive a.
  pyruvate-kinase deficiency a.
  a. refractoria sideroblastica
  refractory a.
  refractory a. with hyperplastic bone marrow
  refractory normoblastic a.
  refractory sideroblastic a.
  renal a.
  runner's a.
  secondary a.
  secondary cold antibody autoimmune hemolytic a.
  secondary sideroblastic a.

ane·mia *(continued)*
  sickle cell a.
  sickle cell hemolytic a.
  sideroachrestic a.
  sideroblastic a.
  sideropenic a.
  spherocytic a.
  simple chronic a.
  spur-cell a.
  target cell a.
  thalassemia major hemolytic a.
  thalassemia minor hemolytic a.
  toxic hemolytic a.
  tropical macrocytic a.
  vitamin deficiency megaloblastic a.
  vitamin E–responsive hemolytic a.
  warm antibody autoimmune hemolytic a.
  X-linked hypochromic a.
  X-linked sideroblastic a.

ane·mic

An·er·gan

an·er·gia

an·er·gic

an·er·gy

an·eryth·ro·pla·sia

an·eryth·ro·plas·tic

an·eryth·ro·poi·e·sis

an·eryth·ro·re·gen·er·a·tive

an·eu·ploid

an·eu·ploi·dy

an·eu·rysm

an·gi·na
  agranulocytic a.
  neutropenic a.
  Schultz's a.

an·gio·blas·to·ma

an·gio·cav·er·nous

an·gio·chon·dro·ma

an·gio·dys·tro·phia
    a. ovarii

an·gio·dys·tro·phy

an·gio·el·e·phan·ti·a·sis

an·gio·en·do·the·li·o·ma

an·gio·fi·bro·ma

an·gio·gen·e·sis
    tumor a.

an·gio·gli·o·ma

an·gio·gli·o·ma·to·sis

an·gio·gran·u·lo·ma

an·gi·og·ra·phy

an·gio·he·mo·phil·ia

an·gio·im·mu·no·blas·tic

an·gio·in·farc·tion

an·gio·ker·a·to·ma
    a. corporis diffusum

an·gio·leio·my·o·ma

an·gio·li·po·leio·my·o·ma

an·gio·li·po·ma

an·gio·lym·phan·gi·o·ma

an·gi·o·ma
    a. arteriale racemosum
    a. cavernosum
    cavernous a.
    a. cutis
    fissural a.
    hypertrophic a.
    a. lymphaticum
    plexiform a.
    simple a.
    telangiectatic a.

an·gi·o·ma·to·sis

an·gi·om·a·tous

an·gio·meg·a·ly

an·gio·myo·li·po·ma

an·gio·my·o·ma

an·gio·myo·sar·co·ma

an·gio·myx·o·ma

an·gio·neo·plasm

an·gio·re·tic·u·lo·en·do·the·
    li·o·ma

an·gio·sar·co·ma

an·gio·ten·sin

an·gio·ten·sin-con·vert·ing
    en·zyme

an·gle
    cerebellopontile a.
    cerebellopontine a.

an·gui·dine

an·irid·ia
    a.–Wilms tumor associa-
    tion

an·iso·chro·ma·sia

an·iso·chro·mia

an·iso·cy·to·sis

an·iso·poi·ki·lo·cy·to·sis

an·ky·rin

3-an·ky·rin

ANLL
    acute nonlymphocytic leu-
    kemia

Ann Ar·bor clas·si·fi·ca·tion
    (for Hodgkin's disease)

Ann Ar·bor stag·ing (for
    Hodgkin's disease)

an·nex·in

an·nu·lar

ano·chro·ma·sia

anom·a·ly
    Alder's a.

anom·a·ly *(continued)*
    Alder's constitutional
        granulation a.
    Alder-Reilly a.
    Chédiak-Higashi a.
    Chédiak-Steinbrinck-Hi-
        gashi a.
    May-Hegglin a.
    Pelger's nuclear a.
    Pelger-Huët a.
    Pelger-Huët nuclear a.
    pseudo–Pelger-Huët a.
    Riedel's a.
    Undritz a.

an·orex·ia
    Heinz body hemolytic a.
    paraneoplastic a.

AN-Sul·fur Col·loid

An·ta-Gel

An·ta·Gel-II

an·tag·o·nist
    folic acid a.
    serotonin a.
    vitamin K a.

An·ta·zone

an·te·ce·dent
    plasma thromboplastin a.
        (PTA)

an·tho·cy·a·nin·emia

an·thra·cene

an·thra·cy·cline

an·ti·ag·glu·ti·nin

an·ti·ana·phy·lax·is

an·ti·an·ti·bo·dy

an·ti·an·ti·tox·in

an·ti·au·tol·y·sin

an·ti·bi·ot·ic
    antitumor a's
    athracycline a's

an·ti·blas·tic

an·ti·body
    anaphylactic a.
    anticardiolipin a.
    anti-D a.
    anti-idiotype a.
    anti-idiotypic a.
    antimelanoma a.
        XMMME-001-TRA
    anti-μ a.
    antineuroblastoma a's
    antinuclear a's (ANA)
    antiphosphoid a.
    antiphospholipid a.
    antiplatelet a.
    antitumor a's
    autoantiidiotypic a's
    autologous a.
    bispecific a.
    blocking a.
    CAMPATH-1 a.
    CD a.
    cell-bound a.
    cell-fixed a.
    cold a.
    cold-reactive a.
    complement-fixing a.
    complete a.
    cross-reacting a.
    cytophilic a.
    cytotoxic a.
    cytotropic a.
    Donath-Landsteiner a.
    DREG a.
    human antimouse a.
        (HAMA)
    immune a.
    incomplete a.
    indium In 111 antimelan-
        oma a. XMMME-0001-
        DTPA
    indium In 111 murine
        anti-CEA monoclonal a.
        ZCE 025
    indium In 111 murine
        monoclonal a. B72.3

an·ti·body *(continued)*
 iodine I 131 Lym-1 mono-
  clonal a.
 iodine I 131 murine monoclonal a. IgG$_{2a}$
 isophil a.
 monoclonal a's
 monoclonal a. 17-1A
 monoclonal a's PM-81 and
  AML-2-23
 natural a's
 polyclonal a.,
 radiolabeled a.
 Rh a's
 saline a.
 sensitizing a.
 trump a.
 warm a.
 warm-reactive a.

an·ti·body-de·pen·dent

an·ti·can·cer

an·ti·cho·les·ter·emic

an·ti·cho·les·te·rol·emic

an·ti·cho·lin·er·gic

an·ti·co·ag·u·lant
 circulating a.
 coumarin a's
 endogenous a.
 heparin-like a.
 lupus a.
 oral a.

an·ti·co·ag·u·la·tion

an·ti·co·ag·u·la·tive

an·ti·co·ag·u·lin

an·ti·com·ple·ment

an·ti·com·ple·men·ta·ry

an·ti·con·vul·sant

an·ti-D

an·ti·emet·ic

an·ti·es·tro·gen
 antitumor a.

an·ti·fi·bri·nol·y·sin

an·ti·fi·bri·no·lyt·ic

An·ti·flux

an·ti·fo·late

an·ti·gen
 allogeneic a.
 B a.
 B-cell a.
 blood-group a's *(see Appendix I)*
 carcinoembryonic a. (CEA)
 cell surface a.
 Chido a.
 class I a's
 class II a's
 class III a's
 common a.
 common acute lympho-
  blastic leukemia a.
  (CALLA)
 common chronic lympho-
  cytic leukemia (CLL) a.
  (cCLLa)
 common CLL a. (cCLLa)
 common leukocyte a's
 complete a.
 conjugated a.
 cross-reacting a.
 D a.
 DREG a.
 E a.
 early a.
 Epstein-Barr nuclear a.
 Factor VIII coagulant a.
  (VIIIcag)
 Factor VIII–related a.
  (Factor VIIIag)
 fetal tumor-associated a's
 H a.
 H-2 a's
 heterogeneic a.
 heterogenetic a.
 heterologous a.

an·ti·gen *(continued)*
    heterophil a.
    heterophile a.
    histocompatibility a's
    histocompatibility a's, ma-
      jor
    histocompatibility a's, mi-
      nor
    HLA a's *(see Appendix 2)*
    HLA D-region a.
    homologous a.
    human leukocyte a.
    H-Y a.
    Ia a.
    I/i a.
    isogeneic a.
    isophile a.
    leukocyte common a.
    lymphocyte a.
    lymphocyte-defined (LD)
      a's
    lymphocyte func-
      tion–associated a.
    major histocompatibility a.
    membrane a.
    minor histocompatibility
      a.
    Mo3 a.
    neutrophil specifc a.
    oncofetal a.
    organ-specific a.
    Oz a.
    pan–B cell a.
    pancreatic oncofetal a.
      (POA)
    partial a.
    private a's
    proliferating cell nuclear
      a. (PCNA)
    proliferation a.
    prostate-specific a.
    public a's
    SD a's
    self-a.
    sero-defined (SD) a's
    serologically defined (SD)
      a's
    Sr-a platelet a.

an·ti·gen *(continued)*
    T a.
    Tac a.
    T-cell a.
    T cell cytoplasmic a.
    T-dependent a.
    T-independent a.
    tissue-specific a.
    transplantation a's
    tumor a.
    tumor-associated a.
    tumor-specific a. (TSA)
    tumor-specific transplanta-
      tion a. (TSTA)
    VLA a.
    xenogeneic a.

an·ti·gen·emia

an·ti·gen·emic

an·ti·gen·ic

an·ti·ge·nic·i·ty

an·ti·glob·u·lin

an·ti·he·mag·glu·ti·nin

an·ti·he·mol·y·sin

an·ti·he·mo·lyt·ic

an·ti·he·mo·phil·ic

an·ti·his·ta·mine

an·ti-id·io·type

an·ti·leu·ko·cyt·ic

an·ti·lew·is·ite
    British a. (BAL)

an·ti·me·tab·o·lite

an·ti·nau·se·ant

an·ti·neo·plas·tic

an·ti·neo·plas·ton

an·ti·on·co·gene

an·ti·on·cot·ic

an·ti·pha·go·cyt·ic

an·ti·plas·min
  α_1-a.
  α_2-a.

an·ti·plas·tic

an·ti·plate·let

an·ti·pro·throm·bin

an·ti·sense

an·ti·se·rum
  common acute lympho-
    blastic leukemia anti-
    serum (CALLA)

an·ti·sta·sin

an·ti·throm·bin
  a. I
  a. III
  a. III *Pittsburgh*

an·ti·throm·bo·plas·tin

an·ti·throm·bot·ic

an·ti·thy·mo·cyte

α_2-an·ti·tryp·sin

an·ti·tu·mor·i·gen·ic

An·tu·ran

An·tu·rane *(US)*

An·xan·il

AP
  adenomatous polyp

APC
  adenomatous polyposis coli

AP1 fac·tor

aph·e·re·sis

aphi·di·co·lin

apla·sia
  acquired pure red cell a.
  bone marrow a.
  chronic constitutional red
    cell a.
  congenital pure red cell a.

apla·sia *(continued)*
  constitutional red cell a.
  pure red cell a.
  pure white cell a.
  red cell a.

APO
  doxorubicin, prednisone,
    vincristine, and 6-mer-
    captopurine, asparagi-
    nase, and methotrexate

Apo-Ci·met·i·dine

Apo-Di·py·rid·a·mole

Apo-Hy·droxy·zine

Apo-K

apo·lipo·pro·tein

Apo-Per·phen·a·zine

ap·op·to·sis

Apo-Ra·ni·ti·dine

Apo-Sul·fin·py·ra·zone

Apo-Tol·bu·ta·mide

apo·trans·fer·rin

Apo-Tri·a·zide

ap·pa·rat·us *pl.* ap·pa·rat·
  us, ap·pa·rat·us·es
  Abbé-Zeiss a.
  Barcroft's a.
  Tiselius a.

ap·pear·ance
  histologic a.
  onion-skin a. of bone
  sunburst a.

apro·ti·nin

Apt
  A. test

APUD
  amine precursor uptake
    and decarboxylation

apud·o·ma

Aq·ua·MEPH·Y·TON

ara-C
  cytarabine
  cytosine arabinoside

arach·i·don·ate

arach·i·don·ic acid

Ar·a·len

ARC
  AIDS-related complex

area *pl.* areae, areas
  B-dependent a.
  body surface a.
  T-dependent a.
  thymus-dependent a.
  thymus-independent a.
  T-independent a.

are·gen·er·a·tive

are·o·la *pl.* are·o·lae

are·o·lar

ARF
  acute renal failure

ar·ga·tro·ban

ar·gent·af·fin·i·ty

ar·gen·taf·fi·no·ma
  a. of bronchus

ar·gi·di·pine

ar·gi·nase

ar·gi·nine
  a. vasopressin

ar·gi·ni·no·suc·cin·ic·ac·i·
  de·mia

ar·gyr·emia

ar·gy·ro·phil·ia

ar·gy·ro·phil·ic

Ar·neth
  A's classification
  A. count

Ar·neth *(continued)*
  A's formula
  A. index

ar·rest
  G_0-G_1 a.
  maturation a.

Ar·res·tin

ar·rhe·no·blas·to·ma

ar·rhe·no·ma

Ar·row catheter

ar·se·nic

ar·sine

ar·te·ri·og·ra·phy
  CT a.

ar·te·ry
  hepatic a.

ar·thri·tis *pl.* ar·thrit·i·des
  hemophilic a.
  paraneoplastic a.

Ar·tic·u·lose-50

ar·ti·fact
  crush a.

ary·ep·i·glot·tic

ar·yl·sul·fa·tase B (ARSB)
  deficiency

ar·y·te·noid

as·bes·tos

as·ci·tes
  chylous a.
  malignant a.

ASCO
  American Society of Clinical Oncology

as·cor·be·mia

as·cor·bic acid

ASP
  L-asparaginase

Asp
   L-asparaginase

L-ASP
   L-asparaginase

L-Asp
   L-asparaginase

as·par·a·gin·ase
   L-a.

as·pect

as·pi·ra·tion
   bone marrow a.
   fine-needle a.
   needle a.

as·pi·rin
   buffered a.
   a., sodium bicarbonate,
     and citric acid

as·say
   antithrombin III–heparin
     cofactor a.
   binding a.
   blastogenesis a.
   cell-mediated lympholysis
     (CML) a.
   CHD_{50} a.
   clonogenic a.
   color complementation a.
   complement a., hemolytic
   complement a., total
   complement a., whole
   DNA transformation a.
   dye exclusion a.
   E rosette a.
   EAC rosette a.
   enzyme-linked immuno-
     sorbent a.
   fibrin plate a.
   fibrinogen a.
   four-point a.
   hemagglutination inhibi-
     tion (HI, HAI) a.
   hemolytic plaque a.
   hormonal a.
   immune a.

as·say *(continued)*
   immune adherence hem-
     agglutination a. (IAHA)
   immunobead a.
   immunoradiometric a.
   Jerne plaque a.
   Limulus amebocyte a.
   lymphocyte proliferation a.
   microcytotoxicity a.
   microencapsulation a.
   mobility shift a.
   radioligand a.
   radioreceptor a.
   Raji cell a.
   stem cell a.

as·so·ci·a·tion
   aniridia–Wilms tumor a.

as·tem·i·zole

Ast·ler-Col·ler
   A-C. staging (for colorectal
     carcinoma)

ASTR
   American Society for
     Therapeutic Radiology

as·tro·blas·to·ma

as·tro·cyte
   fibrillary a.
   gemistocytic a.
   pilocytic a.
   protoplasmic a's

as·tro·cy·to·ma
   anaplastic a.
   cerebellar a.
   cerebral a.
   cystic cerebellar a.
   a. fibrillare
   fibrillary a.
   gemistocytic a.
   juvenile pilocytic a.
   mixed a.
   pilocytic a.
   a. protoplasmaticum
   protoplasmic a.

ASX
    asymptomatic

asyn·cli·tism

AT-III
    antithrombin III

Ata·rax

atax·ia
    a.-telangiectasia

ATP
    adenosine triphosphate

atrans·fer·ri·ne·mia

At·ro·mid·S

at·ro·phy
    reversionary a.

At·rox·in

atyp·ia
    cellular a.

Au-an·ti·gen·emia

Au·ber·ger
    A. blood group

AuBMT
    autologous bone marrow
      transplantation

au·di·om·e·try

Au·er
    A. body
    A. rod

au·ta·coid

au·to·ag·glu·ti·na·tion

au·to·ag·glu·ti·nin

au·to·an·ti·bo·dy

au·to·an·ti·com·ple·ment

au·to·an·ti·gen

au·to·body

au·to·crine

au·to·eryth·ro·phago·cy·to·sis

au·to·gen·e·ic

au·tog·e·nous

au·to·graft

au·to·graft·ing
    bone marrow a.

au·to·he·mag·glu·ti·na·tion

au·to·he·mag·glu·ti·nin

au·to·he·mol·y·sin

au·to·he·mol·y·sis

au·to·he·mo·lyt·ic

au·to·he·mo·ther·a·py

au·to·he·mo·trans·fu·sion

au·to·im·mune

au·to·im·mu·ni·ty

au·to·im·mu·ni·za·tion

au·to·isol·y·sin

au·to·leu·ko·ag·glu·ti·nin

au·tol·o·gous

au·tol·y·sate

au·tol·y·sin

au·tol·y·sis

au·to·lyt·ic

au·to·lyze

au·to·nom·ic

au·to·pro·throm·bin
    a. I
    a. II
    a. IIa
    a. C

au·to·ra·di·og·ra·phy

au·to·se·rous

au·to·se·rum

Au·to·sy·ringe pump

au·to·throm·bo·ag·glu·ti·nin

au·to·trans·plant

au·to·trans·plan·ta·tion

AV
   doxorubicin and vincristine

AVAD
   doxorubicin, vincristine, cytarabine, and dexamethasone

avid·i·ty

AVP
   arginine vasopressin

Ax·id

Ayer·za
   A's disease

aza·cy·ti·dine

5-aza·cy·ti·dine

aza·de·oxy·cy·ti·dine

5-AZA-2'-de·oxy·cy·ti·dine

aza·pro·pa·zone

13-aza·pros·ta·no·ic acid

azat·a·dine

aza·thio·prine

az·ide·met·he·mo·glo·bin

az·i·do·thy·mi·dine (AZT)

AZQ
   diaziquone

AZT
   zidovudine (azidothymidine)

Azul·fi·dine

az·ure
   a. A

az·u·ro·phil

az·u·ro·phil·ia

az·u·ro·phil·ic

ba·cille
 b. Calmette-Guérin (BCG)

ba·cil·lus *pl.* ba·cil·li
 Calmette-Guérin b.

BACON
 bleomycin, doxorubicin,
 cyclophosphamide, vin-
 cristine, and mechlorethamine
 bleomycin, doxorubicin, lomustine, vincristine, and
 mechlorethamine

BACOP
 bleomycin, doxorubicin,
 cyclophosphamide, vin-
 cristine, and prednisone

Bac·te·roi·des
 B. fragilis
 B. gingivalis

Bac·trim DS

Bak a/Bak b alloantigen
 system

BAL
 British antilewisite
 acid-base b.

BALT
 bronchial-associated lymphoid tissue

Bal·ti·more Can·cer Re·
 search Cen·ter

Bam·ber·ger
 B's hematogenic albumin-
 uria

ban·din

band·ing
 G-b.
 Giemsa b.
 reverse b.

BAPP
 bleomycin, doxorubicin,
 cisplatin, and prednisone

Bar·croft
 B's apparatus

bar·i·um
 b. hydroxide

Barr
 Epstein-B. nuclear antigen
 Epstein-B. virus

Bar·rett
 B's esophagus

Bart
 B's hemoglobin

Bar·tho·lin
 B's gland

Bar·to·nel·la
 B. anemia

bar·to·nel·lo·sis

Bart·ter
 B's syndrome

ba·sa·loid

ba·sa·lo·ma

base
 b. pair

base·line

ba·sis ipl.ba·ses
 molecular b.

ba·so·phil

ba·so·phil·ia
 paraneoplastic b.

ba·so·phil·ic

ba·soph·i·lism
 Cushing's b.
 pituitary b.

ba·so·philo·pe·nia

ba·tan·o·pride

Baum·gart·ner
B. perfusion method

B-BPA
B cell–derived burst promoting activity

BC
bleomycin and lomustine

B-CAVe
bleomycin, lomustine, doxorubicin, and vinblastine

BCD
bleomycin sulfate, cyclophosphamide, and dactinomycin

BCDT
bolus dynamic computed tomography

B cell
bone marrow or bursa of Fabricius derived cell

BCG
bacille Calmette-Guérin

BCGF
B cell growth factors

bcl-1 gene

bcl-2 gene

BCNT
boron neutron capture therapy

BCNU
carmustine

Bcnu
carmustine

BCOP
carmustine, cyclophosphamide, vincristine, and prednisone

bcr
breakpoint cluster region

bcr-abl fusion gene

BCRC
Baltimore Cancer Research Center

bcr gene

BCTF
Breast Cancer Task Force

BCVPP
carmustine, cyclophosphamide, vinblastine, procarbazine, and prednisone

BCVPP-Bleo
carmustine, cyclophosphamide, vinblastine, procarbazine, prednisone, and bleomycin sulfate

BCZ-91 (stem cell) line

B-DOPA
bleomycin, dacarbazine, vincristine, and prednisone
bleomycin, dacarbazine, vincristine, prednisone, and doxorubicin

BE
barium enema

bead
immunoreactive b.

BEAM
carmustine, etoposide, cytarabine, and melphalan

Beard
B's treatment

Beck·with
    B.-Wiedemann syndrome

BED
    biologically effective dose

bed
    tumor b.

Bé·guez Cé·sar
    B.C. disease

Beh·la
    B's bodies

Bence Jones
    B.J. proteinemia
    B.J. proteinuria

Ben·e·mid

be·nign

Ben·u·ryl

Ben·za·cot

ben·za·mide
    substituted b's

ben·zan·thra·cene

benz[a]·an·thra·cene

ben·zene

ben·zi·dine

benz·ni·da·zole

ben·zo·ate/phen·yl·ac·e·tate

ben·zol

ben·zo[a]py·rene

3,4-benz·py·rene

BEP
    bleomycin sulfate, etopo-
        side, and cisplatin

Ber·en·blum
    B. model of carcinogenesis

Bernard
    B.-Soulier disease
    B.-Soulier syndrome

ber·yl·li·o·sis

ber·yl·li·um

be·ta-car·o·tene

be·ta-glu·cu·ron·i·dase

be·ta-ly·sin

be·ta·meth·a·sone

be·t$_2$-mi·cro·glob·u·lin

be·ta-Mon·tre·al gene

Bethesda
    B. unit

Bet·ke
    Kleihauer-B. test

Bet·nel·an

BFU-E
    burst-forming
        unit–erythroid

bi·car·bo·nate
    intravenous b.

BiCNU

bi·der·mo·ma

bile ac·id

bil·i·a·ry

bi·line·age

bi·lin·eal

bil·i·ru·bin·emia

Bill·roth
    B's disease
    B. procedure

bind·ing

Bi·net
    B. staging system (for
        chronic lymphocytic leu-
        kemia)

Bio-Gan

bio·mark·er

bi·op·sy
- aspiration b.
- bone marrow b.
- core b.
- fine needle b.
- percutaneous b.
- percutaneous fine-needle
  aspiration b.
- percutaneous lung b.
- stereotactic b.
- thin needle b.

bio·ther·a·py

bio·tin·yl·at·ed

bio·trans·for·ma·tion

bi·phe·no·typ·ic

bi·phe·nyl
- polychlorinated b. (PCB)

bi·phos·pho·nate

bis·an·trene

*bis*chlor·eth·yl ni·tro·so·urea

bis·hy·droxy·cou·ma·rin

Bis·marck brown

Bis·o·dol

bi·spe·cif·ic

Black
- B. operation

black
- amido b.
- fat b. HB
- Sudan b. B

Black·fan
- B.-Diamond anemia
- B.-Diamond syndrome
- Diamond-B. anemia
- Diamond-B. syndrome
- Josephs-Diamond-B. syn-
  drome

blad·der

blast
- b. crisis
- b. transformation

blas·tic

blas·to·cy·to·ma

blas·to·gen·e·sis

blas·to·ma *pl.* blas·to·mas,
  blas·to·ma·ta
- pluricentric b.
- unicentric b.

blas·to·ma·toid

blas·to·ma·to·sis

blas·to·ma·tous

blas·to·mo·gen·ic

blas·to·mog·e·nous

bleed·er

bleed·ing
- esophageal variceal b.
- fibrinolytic b.

Blen·ox·ane

BLEO
- bleomycin sulfate

Bleo
- bleomycin sulfate

ble·o·my·cin
- b. sulfate

BL3 (SCA-1$^+$ stem cell) line

block
- autonomic nerve b.

block·ade
- dopamine b.
- Fc receptor b.

block·ing
- mantle field b.
- spinal cord b.

Blöm·back
- B. fraction I-0

blood
    ACD (acid citrate dex-
      trose) whole b.
    arterial b.
    CPD (citrate phosphate
      dextrose) whole b.
    CPDA-1 (citrate phosphate
      dextrose with adenine)
      whole b.
    defibrinated b.
    fecal b.
    laky b.
    occult b.
    peripheral b.
    sludged b.
    venous b.
    whole b.

blood bank

blood group *(see also*
  Appendix 1)
    ABO b. g.
    Auberger b. g.
    Bg b.g.
    Cartwright b. g.
    Colton b.g.
    Cost-Sterling b.g.
    Diego b. g.
    Dombrock b. g.
    Duffy b. g.
    Fisher b.g.
    H b.g.
    high frequency b. g.
    I b. g.
    Ii b.g.
    Kell b. g.
    Kidd b. g.
    Lewis b. g.
    low frequency b. g.
    Lutheran b. g.
    MN b. g.
    MNS b.g.
    MNSs b.g.
    P b. g.
    Rh b. g.
    Sciana b.g.
    Stoltzfus b.g.
    Vel b.g.

blood group *(continued)*
    Wright b.g.
    Xg b.g.

blood plas·ma

blood se·rum

blood stream, blood·stream

blood type

Bloom
    B. syndrome

blot
    Northern b.
    Southern b.
    Western b.

blue
    basic b. 9
    brilliant b., C.
    brilliant cresyl b.
    Evans b.
    fast b.
    fast b. BNN
    methylene b.
    bone marrow transplanta-
      tion

B-*myb* gene

body
    Auer b's
    Behla's b's
    Bence Jones b's
    "bull's eye" b.
    cancer b's
    carotid b.
    ciliary b.
    Deetjen's b's
    demilune b.
    dense b's
    Döhle's b's
    Döhle's inclusion b's
    Dutcher b.
    elementary b.
    fuchsin b's
    Gordon's elementary b.
    granular b.
    Heinz b's

body *(continued)*
 inner b's
 Mott b's
 no-threshold b's
 onion b's
 Pappenheimer b's
 pearly b's
 platelet dense b.
 Plimmer's b's
 psammoma b.
 Russell b's
 threshold b's
 Verocay b's
 Weibel-Palade b.

BOLD
 bleomycin, vincristine, lomustine, and dacarbazine

Bom·bay
 B. phenotype

bom·be·sin

bone
 b. pain

Bone·fos

Bonn
 B. regimen

BOPP
 bleomycin sulfate, vincristine, procarbazine, and
 prednisone

Borch·grev·ink
 B. technique

Bor·det
 B.-Gengou phenomenon

Bor·de·tel·la
 B. pertussis

Bo·ro·life

Bow·en
 B's disease
 B's precancerous dermato-
 sis

bow·en·oid

box
 CAT b.
 TATA b.

BPA
 burst-promoting activity

brachy·ther·a·py
 interstitial b.

brady·ki·nin

Brain Tu·mor Co·op·er·a·
tive Group

Brain Tu·mor Stu·dy Group

bran·chi·o·ma

break·point
 bcr b.
 Mbc-type b.

Breast Can·cer Task Force

bre·fel·din A

Bren·ner
 B. tumor

Bres·low
 B. system (for melanoma
 staging)

Brij 35

Brill
 B.-Symmers disease

Bro·ders
 B. classification
 B. grade
 B. index

bro·mo·de·oxy·uri·dine

brom·phen·ir·amine

bron·chi·al

bron·chos·co·py
 fiberoptic b.
 rigid b.

Brooke
 B's tumor

Bro·vi·ac cath·e·ter

Brown
   B.-Pearce tumor

brown
   Bismarck b.

bru·cel·lo·sis

Bru·ton
   B's agammaglobulinemia
   B's disease

BS-1 (stromal) cell line

BSD
   Bernard-Soulier disease

BSD hy·per·ther·mia sys·tem

BSF-2
   B cell stimulatory factor 2

BSO
   bilateral salpingo-oopho-
      rectomy
   buthione sulfoxamine

bsp
   basophils

BTSG
   Brain Tumor Study Group

buc·cal

Buck·ley
   B's syndrome

BUdR
   bromodeoxyuridine

buf·fer
   acetate b.
   AMP b.
   barbital b.
   citrate phosphate b.
   glycine b.
   Owren's b.
   phosphate b.

buf·fer·ing
   secondary b.

bulk
   tumor b.

bu·met·a·nide

bur·den
   leukemic cell body b.
   tumor b.

Bur·ger
   Ringertz-B. classification
      (for astrocytomas)

Bur·kitt
   B's lymphoma
   B's tumor

bur·sa pl. bur·sae
   b. of Fabricius

burst
   B cell–derived b.
   erythroid b.

burst form·ing unit-eryth·roid

Bur·ton
   B's agammaglobulinemia

Busch·ke
   B.-Löwenstein tumor

bu·se·rel·in

bu·sul·fan

1,4-bu·tane·di·ol di·meth·
   ane·sul·fo·nate

bu·thi·one sul·fox·amine

But·ter
   B's cancer

bu·ty·rate

bu·ty·ro·phe·none

BVDS
   bleomycin sulfate, vinblas-
      tine, doxorubicin, and
      streptozocin

BXL-40 (stromal) cell line

by·pass
   colonic b.
   gastric b.

C (complement)
    C1
    C1q
    C1r
    C1s
    C2
    C2a
    C2b
    C2 kinin
    C3
    C3a
    C3b
    C3d
    C4
    C4a
    C4b
    C5
    C5a
    C5b
    C6
    C7
    C8
    C9

CA
    cancer
    carcinoma
    cyclophosphamide, doxoru-
      bicin

CA 125 (tumor marker)

Cac·chi·one
    De Sanctis-C. syndrome

ca·chec·tic

ca·chec·tin

ca·chex·ia
    cancer c.
    cancerous c.
    paraneoplastic c.

CAD
    lomustine, melphalan, and
      vindesine

cad·mi·um

CAE
    cyclophosphamide, doxoru-
      bicin, and etoposide

CAF
    cyclophosphamide, doxoru-
      bicin, and fluorouracil

caf·fe·ic ac·id phen·eth·yl es·
    ter

CAFT
    cisplatin, doxorubicin,
      5-fluorouracil, and
      tamoxifen

CAG
    Carcinogen Assessment
      Group

cal·ce·mia

cal·cif·e·di·ol

cal·ci·fi·ca·tion
    benign c.
    central c.
    concentric c.
    diffuse c.
    eccentric c.
    laminar c.
    malignant c.
    popcorn c.
    stippled c.

Cal·ci·le·an

Cal·ci·mar

Cal·ci·par·ine

cal·ci·to·nin
    c.-human
    c.-salmon

cal·ci·tri·ol

cal·ci·um
    c. acetate

cal·ci·um *(continued)*
  alumina, magnesia, and c.
    carbonate
  c. carbonate
  c. carbonate and magnesia
  c. carbonate, magnesia,
    and simethicone
  c. carbonate and simethi-
    cone
  c. chloride
  c. citrate
  c. glubionate
  c. gluceptate
  c. gluconate
  c. glycerophosphate and c.
    lactate
  c. lactate
  c. and magnesium carbon-
    ates
  c. pantothenate
  c. phosphate
  simethicone, alumina, c.
    carbonate, and magnesia

cal·ci·um-ac·ti·vat·ed

Cal·der·ol

CALGB
  Cancer and Leukemia
    Group B

CALGB (Cancer and Leukemia
  Group B) toxicity scale

CALLA
  common acute lympho-
    blastic leukemia antigen

Cal·len·der
  C. classification (for uveal
    melanoma)

Cal·li·son
  C's fluid

Cal·mette
  bacille C.-Guérin
  C.-Guérin bacillus (BCG)

cal·mod·u·lin

cal·pain

cal·pro·mo·tin

cal·re·tic·u·lin

cam·era
  gamma c.

CAMP
  cyclophosphamide, doxoru-
    bicin, methotrexate, and
    procarbazine

cAMP
  cyclic adenosine mono-
    phosphate

CAM·PATH 1G

camp·to·the·cin

Can·a·da
  Cronkhite-C. polyp
  Cronkhite-C. syndrome

ca·nal
  anal c.

can·cer
  acinar c.
  acinous c.
  adenoid c.
  adrenal c.
  adrenocortical c.
  alveolar c.
  c. of ampulla of Vater
  anal margin c.
  aniline c.
  apinoid c.
  c. atrophicans
  betel c.
  bile duct c.
  black c.
  bladder c.
  bone c.
  boring c.
  bowel c.
  brain c.
  branchiogenous c.
  breast c.
  buccal mucosal c.
  Butter's c.
  buyo cheek c.

can·cer *(continued)*
- cecal c.
- cellular c.
- cerebral c.
- cerebriform c.
- cervical c.
- chimney-sweeps' c.
- chondroid c.
- claypipe c.
- colloid c.
- colorectal c.
- contact c.
- corset c.
- c. en cuirasse
- cutaneous c.
- cystic c.
- dendritic c.
- c. à deux
- disseminated c.
- duct c.
- dye workers' c.
- encephaloid c.
- endometrial c.
- endothelial c.
- epidermal c.
- epithelial c.
- fallopian tube c.
- familial breast c.
- follicular thyroid c.
- gallbladder c.
- gastric c.
- gastrointestinal c.
- gingival c.
- glandular c.
- glottic c.
- green c.
- hard c.
- hard palate c.
- head and neck c.
- hereditary nonpolyposis colon c.
- hypopharyngeal c.
- c. in situ
- inoperable c.
- intrahepatic biliary c.
- jacket c.
- kang c.
- kangri c.

can·cer *(continued)*
- kidney c.
- large bowel c.
- laryngeal c.
- latent c.
- lip c.
- liver c.
- lobular invasive c.
- lung c.
- maxillary sinus c.
- medullary c.
- medullary thyroid c.
- melanotic c.
- metastatic c.
- c. of mouth
- mule-spinners' c.
- nasal cavity c.
- nasal vestibule c.
- nasopharyngeal c.
- neuroendocrine c.
- non–small-cell lung c.
- nonfixed c.
- obstructing c.
- obstructive colon c.
- occult c.
- oral c.
- oropharyngeal c.
- ovarian c.
- c. of palate
- pancreatic c.
- papillary thyroid c.
- paraffin c.
- paranasal sinus c.
- parathyroid c.
- penile c.
- c. of penis
- periampullary c.
- pharyngeal wall c.
- pineal c.
- pitch-workers' c.
- postcricoid pharyngeal c.
- primary c.
- primary liver c.
- prostate c.
- pyriform sinus c.
- resectable c.
- retrograde c.
- rodent c.

can·cer *(continued)*
   roentgenologist's c.
   salivary gland c.
   scirrhous c.
   second c.
   secondary c.
   site-specific ovarian c.
   skin c.
   small intestine c.
   soft c.
   soft palate c.
   soft tissue c.
   soot c.
   spinal cord c.
   spindle cell c.
   splenic flexure c.
   stomach c.
   subglottal c.
   suture line c.
   synchronous c.
   tar c.
   testicular c.
   thyroid c.
   thyroid gland c.
   tongue c.
   tubal c.
   tubular c.
   urethral c.
   urinary tract c.
   urothelial c.
   uterine c.
   vaginal c.
   villous duct c.
   vocal cord c.
   vulvar c.

can·cer·emia

can·cer·i·ci·dal

can·cer·i·gen·ic

Can·cer and Leu·ke·mia Co·op·er·a·tive Group B

can·cero·ci·dal

can·cer·o·gen·ic

can·cer·ous

can·cer-ul·cer

can·cri·form

can·croid

can·nab·i·noid

can·nu·la
   infusion c.

CAP
   cyclophosphamide, doxoru-
      bicin, and cisplatin

cap
   Luer-Lok c.

ca·pac·i·ty
   tumor heating c.

cap·su·lo·ma

car·bam·i·no·he·mo·glo·bin

carb·he·mo·glo·bin

car·bin·ox·amine

car·bo·he·mia

car·bo·he·mo·glo·bin

car·bon·emia

car·bo·pla·tin

car·bo·prost

car·boxy·he·mo·glo·bin

car·box·y·he·mo·glo·bin·e·mia

γ-car·box·y·la·tion

car·cin·emia

car·cin·o·gen
   epigenetic c.
   genotoxic c.
   occupational c.
   proximate c.
   ultimate c.

Car·cin·o·gen As·sess·ment Group

car·ci·no·gen·e·sis
   chemical c.
   viral c.

car·cin·o·gen·ic

car·ci·no·ge·nic·i·ty

car·ci·noid
  atypical c.

car·ci·nol·y·sis

car·ci·no·lyt·ic

car·ci·no·ma *pl.* car·ci·no·
  mas, car·ci·no·ma·ta
  acinar c.
  acinic cell c.
  acinous c.
  adenocystic c.
  adenoid cystic c.
  c. adenomatosum
  adenosquamous c.
  adrenal c.
  adrenal cortical c.
  c. of adrenal cortex
  alveolar c.
  alveolar cell c.
  anaplastic c.
  apocrine c.
  Bartholin's gland c.
  basal cell c.
  c. basocellulare
  basaloid c.
  basosquamous cell c.
  breast c.
  bronchial c.
  bronchioalveolar c.
  bronchiolar c.
  bronchogenic c.
  cerebriform c.
  cervical c.
  cholangiocellular c.
  chorionic c.
  choroid plexus c.
  clear cell c.
  colloid c.
  comedo c.
  corpus c.
  cribriform c.
  c. en cuirasse
  c. cutaneum
  cylindrical c.

car·ci·no·ma *(continued)*
  cylindrical cell c.
  duct c.
  ductal c.
  ductal c. in situ
  embryonal c.
  endometrial c.
  epidermoid c.
  epithelial c.
  c. epitheliale adenoides
  exophytic c.
  fallopian tube c.
  fibrolamellar hepatocellu-
    lar c.
  c. fibrosum
  follicular c.
  gallbladder c.
  gelatiniform c.
  gelatinous c.
  giant cell c.
  c. gigantocellulare
  glandular c.
  granulosa cell c.
  hair-matrix c.
  hepatocellular c.
  Hürthle cell c.
  hyperfunctioning adrenal
    cortical c.
  hypernephroid c.
  infantile embryonal c.
  infiltrating c.
  infiltrating lobular c.
  inflammatory c.
  c. in situ
  intermediate-cell c.
  intraepidermal c.
  intraepithelial c.
  intramucosal c.
  invasive c.
  inverting c.
  Krompecher's c.
  Kulchitzky-cell c.
  large-cell c.
  c. lenticulare
  lenticular c.
  lobular c.
  lymphoepithelial c.
  c. medullare

car·ci·no·ma *(continued)*
  medullary c.
  medullary thyroid c.
  melanotic c.
  metachronous c.
  micropapillary intraductal
    c.
  moderately differentiated
    neuroendocrine c.
  c. molle
  morpheaform basal cell c.
  morphealike basal cell c.
  mucinous c.
  c. muciparum
  c. mucocellulare
  mucoepidermoid c.
  c. mucosum
  mucous c.
  multifocal c.
  c. myxomatodes
  nasopharyngeal c.
  neuroendocrine c.
  noduloulcerative basal cell
    c.
  oat cell c.
  oat cell c. of esophagus
  oat cell c. of lung
  c. ossificans
  osteoid c.
  ovarian yolk sac c.
  papillary c.
  papillary-cystic c. of pan-
    creas
  papillary squamous cell c.
  periportal c.
  pigmented basal cell c.
  poorly differentiated neu-
    roendocrine c.
  preinvasive c.
  prickle cell c.
  reactive c.
  renal cell c.
  renal cell c. of kidney
  reserve cell c.
  scar c.
  schneiderian c.
  scirrhous c.
  c. scroti

car·ci·no·ma *(continued)*
  sebaceous c.
  serous c.
  signet ring c.
  signet-ring cell c.
  c. simplex
  sinonasal undifferentiated
    c.
  small-cell c.
  small-cell undifferentiated
    c.
  spheroidal cell c.
  spindle cell c.
  c. spongiosum
  squamous c.
  squamous cell c.
  squamous cell c. of esopha-
    gus
  string c.
  superficial basal cell c.
  c. telangiectaticum
  c. telangiectodes
  thyroid medullary c.
  transitional cell c.
  c. tuberosum
  tuberous c.
  tubular c.
  undifferentiated c.
  c. of unknown primary ori-
    gin
  ureteral c.
  urothelial c.
  vaginal c.
  varicoid c.
  verrucous c.
  c. villosum
  vulvar c.
  well-differentiated neuro-
    endocrine c.
  yolk sac c.

car·ci·no·ma·ta

car·ci·nom·a·toid

car·ci·no·ma·to·sis

car·ci·nom·a·tous

car·ci·no·phil·ia

car·ci·no·phil·ic

car·ci·no·sar·co·ma
  embryonal c.
  c. of esophagus

car·ci·no·sis
  miliary c.
  c. pleurae
  pulmonary c.

car·ci·no·stat·ic

car·ci·nous

car·dio·lip·in

car·dio·my·op·a·thy
  anthracycline c.
  anthracycline-induced c.

car·dio·pro·tec·tive

car·dio·tox·ic·i·ty

car·dio·tox·in

car·di·tis
  radiation c.

care
  continuing c.
  palliative c.
  psychosocial c.
  supportive c.

car·mus·tine

ca·rot·e·noid

car·ri·er

car·ti·lage
  arytenoid c.

Cart·wright
  C. blood group

cas·cade
  arachidonic acid c.
  metastatic c.

cat·a·lase

CAT box

cat·e·chol·amine

cath·emo·glo·bin

ca·thep·sin
  c. D
  c. G

cath·e·ter
  Arrow c.
  Broviac c.
  central venous c.
  Centrasil c.
  Chemocath c.
  Davol c.
  double-lumen c.
  Edwards c.
  Groshong c.
  Hemed c.
  Hickman c.
  implantable subcutaneous
    c.
  indwelling c.
  infusion c.
  inside-the-needle c. (INC)
  Intrasil c.
  Leonard c.
  c. occlusion
  over-the-needle c. (ONC)
  percutaneous transhepatic
    c.
  percutaneously inserted
    central c. (PICC)
  plastic c.
  polyethylene c.
  polyurethane c.
  polyvinyl c.
  Quinton c.
  Raaf c.
  right atrial c.
  Silastic c.
  silicone rubber c.
  single-lumen c.
  small-bore c.
  Teflon c.
  Tenckhoff c.
  triple lumen c.
  vascular access c.
  venous c.

cat·ion
  metallic c.

cat·ion·ic

CATS
    combined abdominal
    transsacral resection
    technique

cau·ter·iza·tion

cau·ter·ize

cau·tery

CAV
    cyclophosphamide, doxoru-
    bicin, and vincristine

cav·i·ty
    oral c.

CAVmP
    cyclophosphamide, doxoru-
    bicin, teniposide, and
    prednisone

ca·vog·ra·phy

CAVP
    lomustine, melphalan, eto-
    poside, and prednisone

CBDCA
    carboplatin

CBV
    cyclophosphamide, car-
    mustine, and etoposide

CBVD
    lomustine, bleomycin sul-
    fate, vinblastine, and
    dexamethasone

cCLLa
    common chronic lympho-
    cytic leukemia (CLL)
    antigen

CCNU
    lomustine

Ccnu
    lomustine

CCS
    Cronkhite-Canada syn-
    drome

CCSG
    Children's Cancer Study
    Group

CCVPP
    cyclophosphamide, lomus-
    tine, vinblastine, procar-
    bazine, and prednisone

CD
    cluster designation

CD an·ti·body

CDDP
    cisplatin

cDNA
    complementary DNA

CD no·men·cla·ture

CEA
    carcinoembryonic antigen

CeeNU

CEF
    cyclophosphamide, epirub-
    icin, and 5-fluorouracil

cef·o·per·a·zone

cef·ta·zi·dime

cef·tri·a·xone

Ce·les·tin
    C's tube

Ce·les·tone

ce·li·o·ma

ce·li·os·co·py

cell
    A172 c.
    Abbé-Zeiss counting c.
    activated c.
    adherent lymphokine-acti-
        vated killer (A-LAK) c.
    adventitial c's

cell *(continued)*

    adventitial reticular c.
    alpha c's
    antigen-reactive c's
    antigen-sensitive c's
    APUD c.
    argyrophilic c's
    atypical c.
    B c's
    band c.
    basal c.
    beta c's
    bipolar c.
    bizarre c.
    blast c.
    blood c's
    burr c.
    cameloid c.
    CEM c.
    circulating tumor c.
    clear c's
    clonogenic c.
    CMK c.
    committed c.
    committed T cell
    convoluted T cell
    cord blood stem c.
    COS-1 c.
    COS-7 c.
    counting c.
    c. cycle
    cytokine-induced killer c.
      (CIK)
    cytotoxic T c's
    Dorothy Reed c's
    effector c.
    embryonic c's
    embryonic stem c.
    emigrated c.
    endothelial c.
    epithelioid c's
    erythroid c's
    excretory duct c.
    fascicular c.
    fat c.
    Ferrata's c.
    gametoid c's
    germ c's

cell *(continued)*

    ghost c.
    giant c.
    hairy c.
    hand mirror c.
    HCD-57 c.
    HEL (human erythroleu-
      kemia) c.
    helper c's
    helper T c.
    hematopoietic stem c.
    HIL-3 c.
    HL-60 c.
    Hodgkin's c's
    Hurthle c.
    hypochromic c.
    immature B c.
    immunoblast B c.
    immunoblast T cell
    immunologically compe-
      tent c.
    inflammatory c.
    intercalated duct c.
    J82 c.
    juvenile c.
    K c's
    K562 c.
    K562 erythroleukemia c.
    K562 leukemia c.
    KB c.
    KG-1 c.
    killer c's
    killer T c's
    c. kinetics
    KL-60 c.
    lacunar c.
    LAK c.
    large cleaved c.
    large noncleaved c.
    leukemia c.
    leukemia colony forming c.
      (L-CFC)
    leukemic c.
    L and H c.
    long-term marrow c.
      (LTMC)
    lymph c.
    lymphadenoma c's

cell *(continued)*
    lymphocyte-activated
      killer (LAK) c's
    lymphoid c.
    lymphokine-activated
      killer (LAK) c.
    M1 leukemia c.
    Marchand's c.
    marrow c.
    mast c.
    megakaryocyte progenitor
      c.
    memory c's
    c. migration
    mononuclear c.
    Mott c.
    mycosis c.
    myeloid c.
    myeloma c.
    natural killer c.
    natural killer–like LAK c.
    necrotic c.
    neoplastic c.
    NK c's
    nucleated c.
    nucleated red c.
    nucleated red blood c.
    null c's
    oat c's
    oat-shaped c's
    PA6 c.
    Paget's c.
    pagetoid c.
    peripheral blood null c.
    peripheral blood stem c.
    perithelial c.
    perivascular c's
    pessary c.
    physaliferous c's
    plasma c's
    pleomorphic c's
    pluripotent stem c.
    polychromatic c's
    polychromatophil c's
    polymorphonuclear c.
    popcorn c.
    pre-B c's
    pre-T c.

cell *(continued)*
    progenitor c.
    RA c.
    Raji c's
    red c.
    red blood c.
    Reed c's
    Reed-Sternberg c's
    segmented c.
    seminoma c.
    sensitized c.
    Sézary c.
    shadow c.
    signet-ring c.
    small anaplastic c.
    small cleaved c.
    small noncleaved c.
    smudge c's
    spider c.
    spindle c.
    stab c.
    staff c.
    star c's
    stem c.
    Sternberg's giant c's
    Sternberg-Reed c's
    striated duct c's
    stroma c.
    suppressor c's
    T c's
    Tγ c's
    Thoma-Zeiss counting c.
    thymoma c.
    Tμ c's
    tumor c.
    U266 c.
    U937 c.
    uncommitted T cell
    veil c's
    veiled c's
    veto c's
    virgin B c.
    wandering c's
    white c.
    white blood c.

cell-me·di·at·ed

cel·lu·lar·i·ty
   mixed c.

cel·lu·li·tis
   perirectal c.

ce·lo·the·li·o·ma

CEM
   lomustine, etoposide, and
      methotrexate

CEM cell

Cena-K

Cen·o·late

cen·ter
   Flemming c.
   germinal c.
   reaction c.

Cen·tral On·col·o·gy Group

Cen·tra·sil catheter

cen·tro·mere

CEP
   lomustine, etoposide, and
      prednimustine

ceph·a·lin
   rabbit brain c.

CEPP(B)
   cyclophosphamide, etopo-
      side, procarbazine, and
      prednisone, with or with-
      out bleomycin

CEPPBL
   cyclophosphamide, etopo-
      side, and procarbazine

cer·a·mide

cer·e·bro·ma

ce·ro·ma

Ce·ru·bi·dine

ce·ru·lo·plas·min

cer·vi·cal

cer·vix *pl.* cer·vi·ces
   uterine c.

CESS cell line

ce·ti·e·dil

ce·ti·e·dil cit·rate

CEV
   cyclophosphamide, etopo-
      side, and vincristine

CEVD
   lomustine, etoposide, vin-
      desine, and dexametha-
      sone

Ce·vi·ta

CF
   classical fractionation
   conventional fractionation

c-*fgr* on·co·gene

c-*fms* pro·to·on·co·gene

c-*fos* pro·to·on·co·gene

CFU-C
   colony forming and unit-
      culture

CFU-E
   colony forming unit-ery-
      throid
   colony forming unit-eryth-
      rocyte

CFU-G
   colony forming unit-gran-
      ulocyte

CFU-GM
   colony forming unit-gran-
      ulocyte-macrophage

CFU-M
   colony forming unit-mac-
      rophage

CFU-meg
   colony forming unit-mega-
      karyocyte

CFU-S
  colony forming unit-spleen
  colony forming unit-stem
    cell

CG
  cathepsin G

CGD
  chronic granulomatous
    disease

C6 (glioma) cell line

cGy
  centigray

CHAC
  cyclophosphamide, hexa-
    methylmelamine, doxo-
    rubicin, and carboplatin

chain
  H c.
  heavy c.
  J c.
  κ c.
  kappa c.
  λ c.
  lambda c.
  light c.

chal·one

cham·ber
  Abbé-Zeiss counting c.
  counting c.
  Thoma-Zeiss counting c.
  Zappert's c.

change
  fibrocystic c's

chan·nel
  calcium c.

CHAP
  cyclophosphamide, hexa-
    methylmelamine, doxo-
    rubicin, and cisplatin

CHART
  continuous, hyperfraction-
    ated, accelerated radio-
    therapy

Chauf·fard
  Minkowski-C. syndrome

Che·al·amide

Ché·di·ak
  C.-Higashi anomaly
  C.-Higashi disease
  C.-Higashi syndrome
  C.-Steinbrinck-Higashi
    anomaly

chei·lo·car·ci·no·ma

che·late

che·la·tion

Che·mo·cath catheter

che·mo·dec·to·ma

che·mo·em·bo·li·za·tion

che·mo·hor·mo·nal

che·mo·in·fu·sion

CHE·MO·MATE system

che·mo·pro·tec·tant

che·mo·pro·tec·tion

che·mo·pro·tec·tor

che·mo·ra·di·a·tion

che·mo·sen·si·tiv·i·ty

che·mo·sen·si·tiz·er

che·mo·sur·gery
  Mohs' c.

che·mo·tax·is

che·mo·ther·a·peu·tic

che·mo·ther·a·py
  adjuvant c.
  cancer c.
  combination c.
  concurrent c.

che·mo·ther·a·py *(continued)*
    consolidation c.
    continuous c.
    curative c.
    delayed c.
    emetogenic c.
    external pump c.
    high-dose c.
    hyperthermic infusion c.
    induction c.
    infusion c.
    intensification c.
    intermittent c.
    interrupted c.
    intra-arterial c.
    intra-artery c.
    intraperitoneal c.
    intrathecal c.
    intravenous c.
    intravesical c.
    maintenance c.
    multiagent combination c.
    non–phase-specific c.
    palliative c.
    parenteral c.
    phase-specific c.
    postremission c.
    preemptive c.
    preoperative c.
    presurgical c.
    primary c.
    salvage c.
    single-agent c.
    timed-sequential c.

Ches·a·peake
    hemoglobin C.

chest
    c. wall

Chi·do
    C. antigen

Chil·dren's Can·cer Stu·dy Group

Chil·dren's Can·cer Stu·dy Group stag·ing (for neuroblastoma)

chi·me·ric

chi·mer·ism
    donor type c.

CHIP
    cis-dichloro-trans-dihy-droxy-*bis*-isopropylamine platinum

CHL
    chlorambucil

Chl
    chlorambucil

Chla·myd·ia
    C. trachomatis

chlor·am·bu·cil

chlor·am·phen·i·col

chlor·az·e·pate

chlor·di·az·ep·ox·ide

chlor·emia

chlo·ride
    picryl c.

chlor·naph·a·zine

2-chlo·ro·de·oxy·aden·o·sine

2-chlo·ro-2'-de·oxy·aden·o·sine

chlo·ro·eryth·ro·blas·to·ma

N,N-bis(2-chlo·ro·eth·yl)-2-naph·thyl·amine

chlo·ro·leu·ke·mia

chlo·ro·lym·pho·sar·co·ma

chlo·ro·ma

chlo·ro·my·elo·ma

chlo·ro·quine

chlo·ro·thi·a·zide

chlo·ro·tri·an·i·sene

chlo·ro·zo·to·cin

chlor·phen·ir·amine

chlor·prom·a·zine

CHLVPP
    chlorambucil, vinblastine,
        procarbazine, and predni-
        sone

ChlVPP
    chlorambucil, vinblastine,
        procarbazine, and predni-
        sone

Cho·lac

cho·lan·gio·ad·e·no·ma

cho·lan·gio·car·ci·no·ma

cho·lan·gio·hep·a·to·ma

cho·lan·gi·o·ma

cho·lan·gio·pan·cre·a·tog·
    ra·phy
    endoscopic retrograde c.
        (ERCP)
    retrograde c.

cho·lan·threne

cho·le·cys·tec·to·my

cho·le·cys·ti·tis

cho·le·cys·tos·to·my
    percutaneous c.

cho·led·o·cho·je·ju·nos·to·
    my

cho·le·sta·sis
    congenital c.

cho·le·ste·a·to·ma

cho·les·ter·e·mia

cho·les·ter·in·e·mia

cho·les·tero·gen·e·sis

cho·les·ter·ol

cho·les·ter·ol·emia

cho·les·ty·ra·mine
    acetyl glyceryl ether phos-
        phoryl c.

cho·lin·er·gic

Cho·lox·in

Choly·bar

CHOMP
    cyclophosphamide, vincris-
        tine, doxorubicin, predni-
        sone, and methotrexate

chon·dro·ad·e·no·ma

chon·dro·an·gi·o·ma

chon·dro·blast

chon·dro·blas·tic

chon·dro·blas·to·ma
    benign c.

chon·dro·car·ci·no·ma

chon·dro·cyte

chon·dro·dys·pla·sia
    diaphyseal c., McKusick
        type
    metaphyseal c., McKusick
        type

chon·dro·en·do·the·li·o·ma

chon·dro·fi·bro·ma

chon·droid

chon·dro·li·po·ma

chon·dro·ma
    c. sarcomatosum
    true c.

chon·dro·ma·to·sis

chon·dro·my·o·ma

chon·dro·myx·o·ma

chon·dro·myxo·sar·co·ma

chon·dro·sar·co·ma
    central c.
    clear cell c.
    mesenchymal c.

chon·dro·sar·co·ma·to·sis

chon·dro·sar·co·ma·tous

chon·dros·te·o·ma

CHOP
cyclophosphamide, doxoru-
bicin, vincristine, and
prednisone

CHOP-BLEO
bleomycin, cyclophospha-
mide, doxorubicin, vin-
cristine, and prednisone

CHOP-Bleo
bleomycin, cyclophospha-
mide, doxorubicin, vin-
cristine, and prednisone

cho·ran·gi·o·ma

chor·do·blas·to·ma

chor·do·car·ci·no·ma

chor·do·epi·the·li·o·ma

chor·do·ma
chondroid c.
sacrococcygeal c.

chor·do·sar·co·ma

cho·rio·ad·e·no·ma
c. destruens

cho·rio·an·gio·fi·bro·ma

cho·rio·an·gi·o·ma

cho·rio·blas·to·ma

cho·rio·car·ci·no·ma
esophageal c.
mediastinal c.
ovarian c.

cho·rio·epi·the·li·o·ma
c. malignum

cho·ri·o·ma

cho·ri·on·epi·the·li·o·ma

cho·ris·to·blas·to·ma

cho·ris·to·ma

cho·roid

cho·roi·dal

CHP134 (neuroblastoma) cell
line

Christ·mas
C. disease
C. factor

chro·maf·fi·no·ma
medullary c.

chro·ma·tid
sister c's

chro·ma·tog·ra·phy
adsorption c.
affinity c.
column c.
gas c. (GC)
gas-liquid c. (GLC)
gas-solid c. (GSC)
gel-filtration c.
gel-permeation c.
high-performance liquid c.
high-pressure liquid c.
  (HPLC)
ion-exchange c.
liquid-liquid c.
molecular sieve c.
paper c.
partition c.
thin-layer c. (TLC)

chro·mic phos·phate P 32

Chro·mi·tope

chro·mi·um
hexavalent c.

chro·mo·gran·in
c. A

chro·mo·mere

chro·mom·e·ter

chro·mo·my·cin A3

chro·mo·some
Ph^1 c.
Philadelphia c.

chro·mo·tox·ic

Chron·u·lac

Chu·ru·ki·an
C.-Schenk stain

chy·lan·gi·o·ma

chy·le·mia

chy·lo·mi·cro·ne·mia

chy·lo·tho·rax

chy·lous

CI
    continuous infusion

CIA
    colony-inhibiting activity

Ci·ba·cal·cin

CIDTP
    combined immunodefi-
        ciency with T-cell pre-
        dominance

CIF
    clonal inhibitory factor

CIK
    cytokine-induced killer
        cell

ci·met·i·dine

C1 INH
    C1 inhibitor

cip·ro·flox·a·cin

cir·cum·scribed

cir·rho·sis
    diffuse c.
    macronodular c.

CISCA
    cisplatin, cyclophospha-
        mide, and doxorubicin

cis·pla·tin

cis·pla·tin/MOB
    cisplatin, mitomycin, vin-
        cristine, and bleomycin
        sulfate

cis-plat·i·num

11-*cis*-ret·i·nal

cis-ret·i·no·ic acid

cit·rate

cit·ric acid
    aspirin, sodium bicarbon-
        ate, and c.a.

cit·ro·vor·um

c-*jun* on·co·gene

c-*kit* on·co·gene

Clari·pex

Clar·i·tin

Clark
    C. system (for staging of
        melanoma)

CLAS
    chronic lymphadenopathy
        syndrome

clas·mo·cy·to·ma

clas·si·fi·ca·tion
    amended Sydney c.
    American Joint Commit-
        tee on Cancer c. (for ex-
        traocular melanoma)
    Ann Arbor c. (for Hodg-
        kin's disease)
    Arneth's c.
    Broders' c.
    Callender c. (for uveal
        melanoma)
    Cotswolds c. (for Hodgkin's
        disease)
    Dukes' c.
    FAB (French-American-
        British) c. (for acute lym-
        phoblastic and myeloge-
        nous leukemias)
    Gell and Coombs c.
    Janský's c.
    Kernohan c. (for astrocyto-
        mas)
    McNeer c.
    Moss' c.
    Peters c. (for Hodgkin's
        disease)
    Rappaport c.

clas·si·fi·ca·tion *(continued)*
    Rappaport c. (for non-Hodgkin's lymphoma)
    Ringertz c. (for astrocytomas)
    Rye c. (for Hodgkin's disease)
    St. Anne-Mayo c. (for astrocytomas)
    Shimada c. (for prognostic factors in neuroblastoma)
    Sydney c. (for extraocular melanoma)
    WHO (World Health Organization) c. (for central nervous system cancer)
    WHO (World Health Organization) c. (for colorectal cancer)
    Working Formulation c. (for non-Hodgkin's lymphoma)

clear·ance
    plasma iron c.

clear·ing
    perinuclear c.

clem·as·tine

cli·vus

CLL
    chronic lymphocytic leukemia

clo·a·co·gen·ic

clo·fi·brate

clo·mi·phene

clon·al
    c. expansion

clo·nal·i·ty

clone

clo·ni·dine hy·dro·chlo·ride

clon·ing
    cDNA c.

clon·ing *(continued)*
    subtraction c.

clo·no·gen
    tumor c.

clo·no·gen·ic

clo·no·type

clo·trim·a·zole

Clough
    C. and Richter's syndrome

clo·za·pine

clus·ter
    α globin gene c.

clus·ter de·sig·na·tion

CMED
    cyclophosphamide, methotrexate, etoposide, and dexamethasone

CMF
    cyclophosphamide (Cytoxan), methotrexate and fluorouracil

CMFP
    cyclophosphamide, methotrexate, fluorouracil, and prednisone

CMFPT
    cyclophosphamide, methotrexate, fluorouracil, prednisone, and tamoxifen

CMFVP
    cyclophosphamide, methotrexate, fluorouracil, vincristine and prednisone

CMK cell

CML
    cell-mediated lympholysis
    chronic myelocytic leukemia

C-MOPP
    cyclophosphamide, me-
        chlorethamine, vincris-
        tine, procarbazine, and
        prednisone

CMV
    cisplatin, methotrexate,
        and vinblastine
    cytomegalovirus

c-*myb* on·co·gene

c-*myc* on·co·gene

CNS
    central nervous system

co·ag·glu·ti·na·tion

co·ag·u·la·bil·i·ty

co·ag·u·la·ble

co·ag·u·lant

co·ag·u·late

co·ag·u·la·tion
    blood c.
    diffuse intravascular c.
    disseminated intravascu-
        lar c. (DIC)
    c. factors (I–XIIIa)

co·ag·u·la·tive

co·ag·u·lo·gram

co·ag·u·lop·a·thy
    antibiotic-induced c.
    consumption c.
    consumptive c.
    dilutional c's
    paraneoplastic c.

COAP
    cyclophosphamide, vincris-
        tine, cytarabine, and
        prednisone

coat
    buffy c.

co·bal·a·min

co·balt

COBMAM
    cyclophosphamide, vincris-
        tine, bleomycin, metho-
        trexate, doxorubicin, and
        semustine

co·car·cin·o·gen

co·car·cino·gen·e·sis

Cod·man
    C's tumor

co·ef·fi·cient
    volume c.

co·fac·tor
    heparin c. II
    platelet c. 1
    platelet c. 2
    platelet c. I
    platelet c. II
    ristocetin c.

COG
    Central Oncology Group

Cohn
    C. fraction I

Cohn·heim
    C's theory

coil
    induction c.

col·chi·cine

Cold·man
    Goldie-C. hypothesis

Cole
    Hopkins-C. reaction

co·lec·to·my
    right c.
    subtotal c.
    total abdominal c.

Co·les·tid

co·les·ti·pol

co·li·tis *pl.* co·lit·i·des
  granulomatous c.
  ulcerative c.

col·la·gen
  birefringent c.

col·la·gen·ase

Col·lin
  C's law

co·lo·anal

co·lon

col·o·ni·za·tion

co·lono·scop·ic

co·lo·nos·co·py

co·lo·rec·tal

col·or·im·e·ter

col·or·i·met·ric

co·los·to·my

Com·az·ol

COMB
  cyclophosphamide, vincris-
    tine, semustine, and
    bleomycin

Com·bi·pres

com·e·do·car·ci·no·ma

COMLA
  cyclophosphamide, vincris-
    tine, methotreate, cytar-
    abine

com·pat·i·ble

Com·pa-Z

Com·pa·zine

com·pe·tence
  immunologic c.

com·pe·ti·tion
  antigenic c.

com·ple·ment (*see also* C)

com·ple·sta·tin

com·plex
  AIDS-related c. (ARC)
  antigen-antibody c.
  circulating immune c.
  H-2 c.
  hapten-carrier c.
  HLA c.
  immune c.
  kallikrein-$\overline{C}$i-inhibitor c.
  major histocompatibility c.
    (MHC)
  membrane attack c.
    (MAC)
  plasmin-antiplasmin c.

com·po·nent
  blood c.
  complement c's
  c's of complement
  extensive intraductal c.
  M c.
  plasma thromboplastin c.
    (PTC)
  secretory c. (SC)

com·pound
  N-nitroso c.

com·pres·sion
  spinal cord c.

ConA
  concanavalin A

con·ca·nav·a·lin A

con·cen·trate
  platelet c's
  prothrombin-complex c.

con·di·tion
  precancerous c.

con·di·tion·ing
  pre-BMT (pre–bone mar-
    row transplantation) c.

con·glu·ti·na·tion

con·glu·ti·nin
  immune c.

con·glu·ti·no·gen

con·iza·tion
  cervical c.

con·ju·gate
  antibody c.
  MoAb c.
  therapeutic c.

con·junc·ti·va *pl.* con·junc·ti·vae

Conn
  C's syndrome

Con·sti·lac

con·stric·tive

Con·stu·lose

con·tinu·ing care

con·trast
  intravenous c.

con·ver·tase
  C3 c.
  C3 proactivator c.
    (C3PAase)
  C5 c.

con·ver·tin

con·vex·i·ty
  cerebral c.

Coo·ley
  C's anemia
  C's disease

Coombs
  Gell and C. classification

Coop·er
  C. regimen

COP
  cyclophosphamide, vincris-
    tine, and prednisone

COPA
  cyclophosphamide, vincris-
    tine, prednisone, and
    doxorubicin

COP-BCNU
  cyclophosphamide, vincris-
    tine, prednisone, and car-
    mustine

COP-BLAM
  cyclophosphamide, vincris-
    tine, prednisone, bleomy-
    cin, doxorubicin, and pro-
    carbazine

COPP
  cyclophosphamide, vincris-
    tine, prednisone, and
    procarbazine

cop·per
  c. nitrate

co·pre·cip·i·tin

cop·ro·por·phy·ria

cop·ro·por·phy·rin

cord
  vocal c.

cor·dot·o·my

Cor·med pump

Cor·med II pump

Cor·med III pump

Cots·wolds clas·si·fi·ca·tion
  (for Hodgkin's disease)

cor·pus·cle
  blood c's
  blood c., red
  blood c., white
  dust c's
  Hassall's c's
  Norris' c's
  pessary c.
  red c.
  reticulated c's
  white c.

Cor·tef

Cor·ten·e·ma

cor·tex *pl.* cor·ti·ces
  adrenal c.

Cor·throp·hin-Zinc

cor·ti·co·ster·oid
  antitumor c's

cor·ti·co·tro·pin

Cor·ti·foam

cor·ti·sone

Cor·y·ne·bac·te·ri·um
  C. parvum

COS-1 cell

COS-7 cell

Cos·me·gen

co·throm·bo·plas·tin

Co·tran·zine

Coulter
  C. counter

count
  Arneth c.
  blood c.
  complete blood c.
  differential c.
  direct platelet c.
  filament-nonfilament c.
  indirect platelet c.
  leukocyte c.
  nadir peripheral blood c.
  neutrophil lobe c.
  platelet c.
  white blood cell c.

coun·ter
  Coulter c.

coun·ter·elec·tro·pho·re·sis

coun·ter·flow

coun·ter·im·mu·no·elec·tro·pho·re·sis

Cowden
  C's disease

CP
  cyclophosphamide and
    prednisone

C3PA
  C3 proactivator

C3PAase
  C3 proactivator convertase

CPD (citrate phosphate
  dextrose) whole blood

CPDA-1 (citrate phosphate
  dextrose with adenine)
  whole blood

CPT
  choroid plexus tumor

CR
  complete remission
  complete response

c-*raf* pro·to·on·co·gene

cra·nio·pha·ryn·gi·o·ma

cra·ni·ot·o·my

c-*ras* pro·to·on·co·gene

cras·sa·men·tum

CRC
  colorectal cancer

cream
  leukocytic c.

C_H region

C_L region

Cre·mo·phor

cre·na·tion

cre·no·cyte

cre·no·cy·to·sis

cren·u·la·tion

cre·o·sote

cri·sis *pl.* cri·ses
  anaphylactoid c.
  aplastic c.

cri·sis *(continued)*
>   blast c.
>   blastic c.
>   deglobulinization c.
>   hypoplastic c.
>   lymphoid blast c.
>   myeloid blast c.
>   splenic sequestration c.

CRM
>   cross-reacting antigenic
>   material
>   cross-reacting material
>   cross-reaction material

CRM +
>   positive for cross-reacting
>   antigenic material
>   positive for cross-reacting
>   material

CRM −
>   negative for cross-reacting
>   antigenic material
>   negative for cross-reacting
>   material

CRM^R
>   cross-reacting antigenic
>   material–reduced
>   cross-reacting mate-
>   rial–reduced

CRM-R
>   cross-reacting antigenic
>   material–reduced

Cronk·hite
>   C.-Canada polyp
>   C.-Canada syndrome

cross-link·ing
>   fibrin c.-l.

cross·match

cross·match·ing

cross-re·ac·tion
>   c.-r. material CRM

cross-reactive

cross-re·ac·tiv·i·ty

cross-re·sis·tance

cross-re·sis·tant

cross-sen·si·ti·za·tion

Cro·ta·lase

Cru·veil·hier
>   C's plexus

cry·o·fi·brin·o·gen

cryo·fi·brin·o·gen·emia

cryo·gam·ma·glob·u·lin

cryo·glob·u·lin

cryo·glob·u·lin·emia

cryo·pre·cip·i·ta·bil·i·ty

cryo·pre·cip·i·tate

cryo·pre·cip·i·ta·tion

cryo·pres·er·va·tion

cryo·pro·tec·tive

cryo·pro·tein

cryo·su·per·na·tant

cryo·sur·gery

cryo·ther·a·py

cryp·to·de·ter·min·ant

crys·tal
>   blood c's
>   Teichmann's c's
>   Virchow's c's

CS
>   clinical stage
>   clinical state
>   conservative surgery

CSA
>   colony-stimulating activity

CSF
>   colony-stimulating factor
>   multi-CSF

CSF-1
   macrophage colony-stimu-
      lating factor

CT
   chemotherapy
   computed tomography

CT-A
   computed tomographic ar-
      teriography

CTAP
   connective tissue activat-
      ing peptide

CT-AP
   computed tomographic ar-
      terial portography

CTCL
   cutaneous T-cell lym-
      phoma

CTL
   cytotoxic T lymphocytes

CTX
   Cytoxan

CTZ
   chemoreceptor trigger zone

cul·ture
   bone marrow c.
   long-term bone marrow c.
   long-term marrow c.
   mixed lymphocyte c.
      (MLC)

cu·pre·mia

cur·abil·i·ty

cu·ret·tage

cur·rent
   axial c.

Cur·re·tab

curve
   dose-response c.
   Price-Jones c.
   survival c.

Cush·ing
   C's basophilism
   C's disease
   C's syndrome
   C's syndrome medicamen-
      tosus

Cu·tait
   Turnbull-C. operation

CVAD
   cyclophosphamide, vincris-
      tine, doxorubicin, and
      dexamethasone

CVB
   lomustine, vinblastine,
      and bleomycin

CVP
   cyclophosphamide, vincris-
      tine, and prednisone

CVPP
   cyclophosphamide, vin-
      blastine, procarbazine,
      and prednisone

CY
   cyclophosphamide

cy·an·he·mo·glo·bin

cy·an·met·he·mo·glo·bin

cy·an·met·myo·glo·bin

cy·a·no·co·bal·a·min
   c. Co 57
   radioactive c.

cy·a·nose

cy·a·nosed

cy·a·no·sis
   central c.
   false c.
   hereditary methemoglobi-
      nemic c.
   peripheral c.

cy·a·not·ic

CYC
  cyclophosphamide

Cyc
  cyclophosphamide

cy·ca·sin

cy·cle
  cell c.
  c. dependence
  division c.
  isohydric c.
  Murphy c. A

cy·clin

cy·cline

cy·clo·cyt·i·dine

Cy·clo·kap·ron

cy·clo·oxy·gen·ase

cyc·lo-oxy·gen·ase de·fic·ien·cy

cy·clo·phos·pha·mide

Cy·clo-Pros·tin

cy·clo·spor·ine

Cy·crin

cyl·in·dro·ma

cy·lin·drom·a·tous

cy·pro·hep·ta·dine

cy·pro·ter·one ac·e·tate

cyst
  aneurysmal bone c.
  craniopharyngeal duct c.
  epidermoid c.
  ovarian c.
  proligerous c.
  pseudomucinous c.
  sebaceous c.
  suprasellar c.

cys·tad·e·no·car·ci·no·ma
  papillary c.
  pseudomucinous c.

cys·tad·e·no·ma
  c. adamantinum
  c. lymphomatosum
  mucinous c.
  papillary c.
  papillary c. lymphomato-
    sum
  pseudomucinous c.
  serous c.

cys·ta·thi·o·nine syn·thase

cys·ta·thi·o·nine β-syn·thase

cys·ta·thi·o·nine syn·thase
  de·fi·cien·cy

cys·ta·tin

cys·tec·to·my
  partial c.
  radical c.

cys·te·ine pro·tein·ase

cys·tin·emia

cys·ti·tis
  radiation c.

cys·to·ad·e·no·ma

cys·to·car·ci·no·ma

cys·to·epi·the·li·o·ma

cys·to·fi·bro·ma

cys·to·ma

cys·to·ma·ti·tis

cys·to·ma·tous

cys·to·pros·ta·tec·to·my

cys·to·sar·co·ma

Cy·ta·dren

cyt·a·phe·re·sis

cy·tar·a·bine
  high-dose c.

Cy/TBI
  cyclophosphamide and
    total body irradiation

cy·the·mol·y·sis

cy·ti·dine
   c. arabinoside

cy·to·ad·he·sin

cy·to·ad·he·sion

cy·to·an·a·ly·zer

cy·to·cen·tri·fuge

cy·to·chal·a·sin
   c. B

cy·to·chem·i·cal

cy·to·chem·is·try

cy·to·chrome
   c. b558
   c. P-450

cy·to·di·ag·no·sis
   exfoliative c.

cy·to·flu·o·rom·e·try

cy·to·gen·e·sis

cy·to·ge·net·ic

cy·to·ge·net·ics

cy·to·glom·er·a·tor

cy·to·ker·a·tin

cy·to·kine
   recombinant c.

cy·to·ki·net·ic

cy·tol·o·gy
   exfoliative c.
   peritoneal c.
   urine c.

cy·tol·y·sate
   blood c.

cy·tol·y·sin

cy·tol·y·sis
   immune c.

cy·to·ma

cy·to·meg·a·lo·vi·rus

Cy·to·mel

cy·tom·e·ter

cy·tom·e·try
   flow c.

cy·to·mor·phol·o·gy

cy·to·pe·nia
   spleen-induced c.

cy·to·phago·cy·to·sis

cy·toph·a·gous

cy·toph·a·gy

cy·to·plasm
   amphophilic c.

cy·to·re·duc·tion

cy·to·re·duc·tive

Cy·to·sar

Cy·to·sar-U

cy·to·sine
   c. arabinoside

Cy·to·spar

cy·to·tox·ic

cy·to·tox·ic·i·ty
   antibody-dependent c.
   antibody-dependent cell-
      mediated c.
   antibody-dependent cellu-
      lar c.
   cell-mediated c.
   immunologic c.

cy·to·tox·in

cy·to·trop·ic

Cy·tox·an

cyVADIC
   cyclophosphamide, vincris-
      tine, doxorubicin, and
      dacarbazine

D
    daunorubicin

DAC
    decitabine

da·car·ba·zine

Da·cron

DACT
    dactinomycin

Dact
    dactinomycin

dac·ti·no·my·cin

dam·age
    diffuse alveolar d.

Da·mi
    D. human megakaryocytic
        cell line

da·na·zol

Dan·los
    Ehlers-D. syndrome

Dan·ysz
    D's phenomenon

Da·rier
    D's disease

Dau·di
    D. cell line

daugh·ter
    radon d's

dau·no·my·cin

dau·no·ru·bi·cin
    d. hydrochloride

Da·vol catheter

DAY·MATE system

DC
    death certificate

DCBE
    double-contrast barium
        enema

DCF
    deoxycoformycin

DCIS
    ductal carcinoma in situ

DDAVP
    desmopressin

ddC
    dideoxycytidine

ddI
    dideoxyinosine

DDP
    cisplatin (*cis*-dichlorodiam-
        mineplatinum II)

Ddp
    cisplatin (*cis*-dichlorodiam-
        mineplatinum II)

DDTC
    diethyldithiocarbamate

death
    cell d.

DEB
    diepoxybutane

deb·ris·o·quine

de·bulk·ing

Dec·a·dron

Deca-Dur·ab·o·lin

de·car·box·y·la·tion

de·cho·les·ter·in·iza·tion

de·cho·les·ter·ol·iza·tion

de·cid·u·o·ma
    d. malignum

de·ci·ta·bine

57

de·co·ag·u·lant

de·com·pres·sion
  biliary d.

de·dif·fer·en·ti·a·tion

Deet·jen
  D's bodies

de·fect
  tumor d.

de·fen·sin

de·fer·ox·amine
  d. mesylate

de·fi·bri·nat·ed

de·fi·bri·na·tion

de·fi·bri·no·gen·a·tion

de·fi·bro·tide

de·fi·cien·cy
  antithrombin III d.
  coagulation factor d.
  cyclooxygenase d.
  factor d.
  factor V d.
  factor VII d.
  factor X d.
  factor XI d.
  factor XII d.
  factor XIII d.
  Fletcher factor d.
  folic acid d.
  heparin cofactor II d.
  IgA d., isolated
  IgA d., selective
  immune d.
  iron d.
  leukocyte adhesion d.
  leukocyte G6PD d.
  α_2 macroglobulin d.
  MPO (myeloperoxidase) d.
  muscle-type phosphofruc-
    tokinase d.
  Passovoy factor d.
  prekallikrein d.
  protein C d.

de·fi·cien·cy *(continued)*
  protein S d.
  purine nucleoside phos-
    phorylase d.
  specific granule d. (SGD)
  vitamin d.
  vitamin K d.

de·form·a·bil·i·ty
  erythrocyte d.
  leukocyte d.

de·for·ma·tion

de·gen·er·a·tion
  basic d.
  basophilic d.
  red d.

De·gos
  D. disease
  D. syndrome

de·gran·u·la·tion

de·hy·dro·epi·an·dros·ter·
  one

Del·ad·i·ol-40

Del·a·lu·tin

Del·a·test

Del·a·tes·tryl

Del·es·tro·gen

de·le·tion
  chromosomal d.
  chromosome d.
  DNA d.

del·le

Del·ta-Cor·tef

del·ta-thal·as·se·mia

Del·tec-Phar·ma·cia CADD
  pump

de·mar·ca·tion

de·meth·oxy·doxo·ru·bi·cin

den·si·tom·e·try
CT d.

den·ti·no·blas·to·ma

den·ti·no·ma

den·ti·nos·te·oid

den·to·ma

de·oxy·aden·o·sine

de·oxy·cho·late

de·oxy·co·for·my·cin

de·oxy·doxo·ru·bi·cin

de·oxy·he·mo·glo·bin

de·oxy-man·no-oc·tu·lo·son·ic acid

de·oxy·myo·glo·bin

de·oxy·ri·bo·nu·cle·ic acid

de·oxy·thio·guan·o·sine

dep·An·dro

de·pen·dence
cell cycle d.

de·ple·tion
leukocyte d.
lymphocyte d.
plasma d.
T cell d.

dep·Med·a·lone

De·po·ject

De·po-Med·rol

De·po·pred

De·po-Pred·ate

De·po·test

De·po-Tes·tos·ter·one

de·pres·sion
d. of bone marrow
bone marrow d.
hematoporphyrin d.

der·ma·tan sul·fate

der·ma·ti·tis *pl.* der·ma·tit·i·des
precancerous d.

der·ma·to·fi·bro·ma

der·ma·to·fi·bro·sar·co·ma
d. protuberans

der·ma·to·my·o·ma

der·ma·to·myo·si·tis
paraneoplastic d.

der·ma·to·sis *pl.* der·ma·to·ses
acute febrile neutrophilic d.
Bowen's precancerous d.
precancerous d.

DES
diethylstilbestrol

Des
diethylstilbestrol

des·ami·no-8-D-ar·gi·nine vaso·pres·sin (DDAVP)

De Sanc·tis
D.-Cacchione syndrome

de·sen·si·ti·za·tion

Des·fer·al
D.-bound iron reagent

des·hy·dre·mia

des·ic·ca·tion

des·ig·na·tion
cluster d.

des·mo·cy·to·ma

des·moid

des·mo·ma

des·mo·neo·plasm

des·mo·pla·sia

des·mo·plas·tic

des·mo·pres·sin

de·sul·fa·to·hi·ru·din

de·ter·mi·nant
    antigenic d.
    hidden d.
    HLA-D restricted d.
    immunogenic d.
    sequential d.

de·ter·mi·na·tion
    estrogen receptor d.

de·to·ru·bi·cin

DETOX

deu·tero·he·min

deu·tero·he·mo·phil·ia

de·vel·op·ment
    clonal d.

de·vi·a·tion
    complement d.
    immune d.
    d. to the left
    d. to the right

de·vice
    cell saver d.

DEX
    dexamethasone

Dex
    dexamethasone

dex·a·meth·a·sone

dex·chlor·phen·ir·a·mine

Dex·ol T.D.

dex·tran
    d. 70

dex·tro·thy·rox·ine

D-fac·tor

DFMO
    difluoromethylornithine

DFS
    disease-free survival

DH
    diffuse histiocytic lym-
        phoma

DHAP
    dexamethasone, high-dose
        cytarabine, and cisplatin

DHEA
    dehydroepiandrosterone

DHL
    diffuse histiocytic lym-
        phoma

DHT
    dihydrotachysterol

di·a·cyl·glyc·er·ol

di·a·graph

4,4′-di·ami·no·bi·phen·yl

Di·a·mond
    Blackfan-D. anemia
    Blackfan-D. syndrome
    D.-Blackfan anemia
    D.-Blackfan syndrome
    Josephs-D.-Blackfan syn-
        drome
    Schwachman-D. syndrome

di·an·hy·dro·ga·lac·ti·tol

o-di·an·isi·dine Di-HCl

Di·a·non

di·a·pe·de·sis

di·a·pe·det·ic

di·a·pi·re·sis

di·ar·rhea
    serotonin-induced d.

di·ar·rhe·o·gen·ic

Dia·stat

di·ath·e·sis
    hemorrhagic d.

Di·a·zide

di·azi·quone

di·az·ox·ide

di·benz·an·thra·cene

di·benz[*a,h*]·an·thra·cene

di·benz-di·bu·tyl an·thra·quin·ol

di·bro·mo·dul·ci·tol

di·bro·mo·man·ni·tol

DIC
    disseminated intravascular coagulation

di·chlo·ral·phen·a·zone

di·chlo·ro·meth·o·trex·ate

dic·ty·o·ma

di·de·oxy·cy·ti·dine

di·de·oxy·ino·sine

di·der·mo·ma

DIDOX

Di·dro·nel

Di·e·go
    D. blood group

di·epoxy·bu·tane (DEB)

di·eth·yl·di·thio·car·ba·mate

di·eth·yl·stil·bes·trol

di·eth·yl sul·fate

dif·fer·en·ti·a·tion
    cell d.
    epithelial d.
    lymphoid d.

dif·fu·sion
    double d.
    double d. in one dimension
    double d. in two dimensions
    gel d.
    single d.
    single radial d.

Di·flu·can

di·flu·o·ro·meth·yl·or·ni·thine (DMFO)

Di·George
    D's syndrome

di·gly·co·al·de·hyde

Di Gu·gliel·mo
    Di G. disease
    Di G. syndrome

di·hem·a·to·por·phy·rin
    d. ethers

di·hy·dro·er·got·amine

di·hy·dro·fo·late

di·hy·dro·tach·ys·te·rol

di·hy·droxy·alu·mi·num
    d. aminoacetate
    d. sodium carbonate

di·iso·pro·pyl flu·o·ro·phos·phate

dik·ty·o·ma

Di·lau·did

di·lu·tion
    limiting d.

di·men·hy·dri·nate

p-di·meth·yl·am·i·no·az·o·ben·zene

7,12-di·meth·yl·benz[*a*]an·thra·cene

di·meth·yl·car·bam·o·yl di·ox·ide

di·meth·yl sulf·ox·ide

di·meth·yl·tri·a·zeno·im·id·az·ole car·box·amide

di·ni·tro·chlo·ro·ben·zene

di·no·prost·one

Di·o·val

di·pep·ti·dyl ami·no·pep·ti·dase

di·phen·hy·dra·mine

di·phen·i·dol

di·phen·yl·pyr·a·line

2,3-di·phos·pho·glyc·er·ate

di·phos·pho·nate

dip·loid

Di·prid·a·cot

di·py·rid·a·mole

DIS
   deiayed iodine scanning

di·sac·cha·ride tri·pep·tide
   glyc·er·ol di·pal·mi·to·yl

dis·ease (see also under
   syndrome)
   allogeneic d.
   alpha chain d.
   alpha heavy chain d.
   autoimmune d.
   Ayerza's d.
   Béguez César d.
   benign breast d.
   Bernard-Soulier d.
   Billroth's d.
   Bowen's d.
   Brill-Symmers d.
   Bruton's d.
   Chédiak-Higashi d.
   Christmas d.
   chronic cold agglutinin d.
   chronic granulomatous d.
      (CGD)
   cold hemagglutinin d.
   combined immunodefi-
      ciency d.
   Cooley's d.
   Cowden's d.
   Cushing's d.
   Darier's d.
   Degos' d.
   delta heavy chain d.

dis·ease *(continued)*
   Di Guglielmo d.
   Duncan's d.
   extensive d.
   Fanconi's d.
   Franklin's d.
   Gaisböck's d.
   gamma chain d.
   gamma heavy chain d.
   Gaucher's d.
   gestational trophoblastic
      d.
   giant platelet d.
   Gilbert's d.
   Glanzmann's d.
   glycogen storage d.
   graft-versus-host (GVH) d.
   Graves' d.
   d. of the Hapsburgs
   heavy-chain d's
   Heckathorn's d.
   hematopoietic neoplastic d.
   hemoglobin d.
   hemoglobin C d.
   hemoglobin C–thalassemia
      d.
   hemoglobin D d.
   hemoglobin E–thalassemia
      d.
   Hers' d.
   Hodgkin's d.
   hydroxylysine-deficient
      collagen d.
   immune-complex d's
   immunodeficiency d.
   inflammatory bowel d.
   Kahler's d.
   Kawasaki d.
   Letterer-Siwe d.
   light chain deposition d.
   limited-stage d.
   local regional d.
   lymphocyte-depleted
      Hodgkin's d.
   lymphocyte-predominant
      Hodgkin's d.
   Marchiafava-Micheli d.
   Mediterranean d.

dis·ease *(continued)*
  metabolic bone d.
  metastatic d.
  microdrepanocytic d.
  minimal residual d.
  mu chain d.
  mu heavy chain d.
  mule spinner's d.
  nodular sclerosing Hodgkin's d.
  Osler's d.
  Osler-Vaquez d.
  Owren's d.
  Paget d.
  Paget's d., extramammary
  Paget's d. of nipple
  Pel-Ebstein d.
  peripheral vascular d.
  polyendocrine autoimmune d.
  Pringle's d.
  pseudo-von Willebrand d.
  Reed-Hodgkin d.
  residual d.
  Schüller's d.
  Schultz's d.
  serum d.
  severe combined immunodeficiency d. (SCID)
  sickle-cell d.
  sickle cell–hemoglobin C d.
  sickle cell–hemoglobin D d.
  sickle cell–thalassemia d.
  stable d.
  Sternberg's d.
  storage pool d.
  Symmers' d.
  thalassemia–sickle cell d.
  transfusion-associated d.
  Vaquez' d.
  Vaquez-Osler d.
  veno-occlusive d. of the liver
  von Willebrand's d.
  von Willebrand's d., type I

dis·ease *(continued)*
  von Willebrand's d., type IIa
  von Willebrand's d., type III
  Werner-Schultz d.

dis·ease-free

dis·ger·mi·no·ma

dis·in·te·grin

disk
  blood d.

di·so·di·um clo·dron·ate tet·ra·hy·drate

dis·or·der
  autoimmune d.
  B cell lymphoproliferative d.
  bleeding d.
  bone marrow d.
  clotting d.
  coagulation d.
  immunodeficiency d.
  myeloproliferative d.
  neutrophil d.
  plasma cell d.
  platelet d.
  stem cell d.
  thrombohemorrhagic d.

Di·so·tate

dis·sec·tion
  axillary d.
  lymph node d.
  pelvic d.
  retroperitoneal lymph node d.

di·suc·cin·im·id·yl su·ber·ate (DSS)

di·sul·fi·ram

di·uret·ic

di·ver·sion
  antigenic d.

di·ver·si·ty
   genomic d.

di·ver·tic·u·li·tis

di·ver·tic·u·lum *pl.* di·ver·
tic·u·la
   esophageal d.

di·vi·cine

DL
   doxorubicin and lomustine

DM
   diffuse mixed histiocytic-
   lymphocytic lymphoma

DML
   diffuse mixed histiocytic-
   lymphocytic lymphoma

DMSO
   dimethyl sulfoxide

DNA (deoxyribonucleic acid)
   complementary DNA
   DNA deletion
   DNA fingerprinting
   minisatellite DNA
   DNA transfection

DNAase
   DNAase footprinting

DNA li·gase

DNA poly·mer·ase

DNA po·lym·er·ase I

DNCB
   dinitrochlorobenzene

DNR
   daunorubicin

Dnr
   daunorubicin

Döh·le
   D. inclusion bodies

do·main
   immunoglobulin d's.

do·main *(continued)*
   negative regulatory d.
   (NRD)
   positive regulatory d. I
   (PRDI)
   positive regulatory d. II
   (PRDII)

Dom·brock
   D. blood group

Do·nath
   D.-Landsteiner antibody

do·nee

do·nor
   blood d.
   general d.
   d. screening
   universal d.

do·pa·mine

Dop·pler
   D. ultrasonography
   D. ultrasound

Dor·o·thy Reed
   D.R. cells

dose
   biologically effective d.
   equianalgesic d.
   extrapolated response d.
   high-d.
   intermediate-d.
   low-d.
   d. modification
   standard-d.

do·sim·e·ter

do·sim·e·try

dos·ing
   circadian d.

Down
   D. syndrome

down·stag·ing

dox·e·pin

dox·i·flu·ri·dine

doxo·ru·bi·cin

dox·yl·amine

DOXO
  doxorubicin

Doxo
  doxorubicin

DP
  diminutive polyp

DPDL
  diffuse poorly differen-
    tiated lymphocytic lym-
    phoma

D-phen·yl·al·a·nyl-L-pro·lyl-
  L-ar·gi·nyl-chlo·ro·meth·yl
  ke·tone (PPACK)

Drab·kin
  D's solution

drain·age
  biliary d.
  percutaneous transhepatic
    biliary d.

drep·a·no·cyte

drep·a·no·cyt·e·mia

drep·a·no·cyt·ic

drep·a·no·cy·to·sis

Dres·bach
  D's syndrome

Drick·a·mer
  D. sequence

drug
  analgesic d.
  anticancer d.
  antiplatelet d.
  antitumor d.

drum·stick

Dru·sen·fie·ber

DS19-Sc9 (erythroleukemia)
  cell line

DTIC
  dacarbazine (dimethyltri-
    azenoimidazole carbox-
    amide)

Dtic
  dacarbazine (dimethyltri-
    azenoimidazole carbox-
    amide)

DTIC-Dome

DU
  diffuse undifferentiated
    lymphoma

du·al·ism

Du·breu·ilh
  circumscribed precancer-
    ous melanosis of D.

duct
  bile d.
  excretory d.

duc·tog·ra·phy

Duf·fy
  D. blood group

Duke
  D's method
  D's test

Dukes
  D. classification

Dun·can
  D's disease

du·od·e·ni·tis

Du·pha·lac

Du·rab·o·lin

Du·ra·gen

Du·ra·lone

Du·ra·lu·tin

Du·ra·test

Du·ra·thate-200

Du·rie
    D.-Salmon staging (for
        myeloma)

dust
    blood d. (of Müller)
    chromatin d.

Dutch·er
    D. body

DVC
    dactinomycin, vincristine,
        and cyclophosphamide

DWDL
    diffuse well-differentiated
        lymphocytic lymphoma

D2XRII (hematopoietic) cell
    line

dy·ad

dye
    d. exclusion assay

Dy·nia
    D. abnormality

dys·cra·sia
    blood d.
    plasma cell d's

dys·em·bry·o·ma

dys·eryth·ro·poi·e·sis

dys·eryth·ro·poi·et·ic

dys·fi·brin·o·gen·emia
    hereditary a.

dys·func·tion
    gonadal d.
    immune d.
    neutrophil actin d. (NAD)

dys·func·tion *(continued)*
    platelet d.
    pulmonary d.
    renal d.
    testicular d.

dys·gam·ma·glob·u·lin·emia

dys·gen·e·sis
    reticular d.

dys·ger·mi·no·ma
    ovarian d.

dys·glob·u·lin·emia

dys·gly·ce·mia

dys·hem·a·to·poi·e·sis

dys·hem·a·to·poi·e·tic

dys·he·mo·poi·e·sis

dys·he·mo·poi·et·ic

dys·he·sion

dys·lipo·pro·tein·emia

dys·my·elo·poi·et·ic

dys·pa·reu·nia

dys·pha·gia
    sideropenic d.

dys·pla·sia

dys·poi·e·sis

dys·pro·te·in·emia

dys·pro·throm·bin·emia
    hereditary h.

dys·tro·phy
    reflex sympathetic d.
    C. fraction I

E

EA
early antigen

EACA
ε-aminocaproic acid

EA-D
early antigen—diffuse

EAM
etoposide, dactinomycin, and methotrexate

EAP
etoposide, doxorubicin, and cisplatin

EA-R
early antigen—restricted

East·ern Co·op·er·a·tive On·col·o·gy Group

EBER
Epstein-Barr encoded RNA

EBNA
Epstein-Barr nuclear antigen (test)

EBRT
external beam radiotherapy

Eb·stein
Pel-E. disease
Pel-E. fever

EBV
Epstein-Barr virus

Ec·ar·in

ec·chon·dro·ma

ec·chon·dro·sis

ec·chor·do·sis phys·a·liph·o·ra

ec·chy·mo·sis *pl.* ec·chy·mo·ses

echi·no·cyte

ech·i·no·sis

Eck·er
E's fluid
Rees and E. diluting fluid
Rees-E. solution

eclamp·sia

ECOG
Eastern Cooperative Oncology Group

Eco Ri frag·ment

E-CSF
erythroid colony stimulating factor

Ec·to-ADP·ase

ec·to·derm

ec·to·der·mal

ec·to·nu·cle·o·ti·dase

ec·tro·pi·on
cervical e.

ED
extensive disease

ede·ma
cerebral e.
peritumoral e.

ed·e·tate
e. disodium

EDF
eosinophil differentiation factor

EDM
endothelium-derived monocyte

Ed·wards
E. catheter

EEA
   end-to-end anastomosis

EF
   extended field (irradiation)

ef·fect
   anticholinergic e.
   Fahraeus-Lindqvist e.
   fetal rubella e's
   graft-versus-leukemia e.
   sanctuary e.

ef·fec·tive·ness
   relative biological e.

ef·fi·ca·cy

ef·fu·sion
   malignant e.
   malignant pleural e.
   pericardial e.
   pleural e.
   postirradiation pleural e.

EFP
   etoposide, fluorouracil, and
      cisplatin

EGB
   eosinophilic granuloma of
      bone

EGF
   epidermal growth factor

EGF-R
   epidermal growth factor
      receptor

egr-1 gene

Eh·lers
   E.-Danlos syndrome

EIC
   extensive intraductal com-
      ponent

ei·co·sa·noid

ei·loid

ELAM-1
   endothelial cell adhesion
      molecule-1

elas·tase (pancreatic)

elas·to·fi·bro·ma
   e. dorsi

elas·to·ma
   juvenile e.

El·di·sine

elec·tro·co·ag·u·la·tion

elec·trode
   capacitative e.

elec·tro·des·ic·ca·tion

elec·tro·di·a·ly·zer

elec·tro·en·ceph·a·log·ra·
   phy

elec·tro·im·mu·no·dif·fu·
   sion

elec·tro·pho·re·sis
   counter e.
   gel e.

elec·tro·pho·ret·ic

el·e·ment
   formed e's (of the blood)
   interferon-stimulated re-
      sponse e.

el·e·va·tion
   amylase e.

el·i·nin

ELISA
   enzyme-linked immuno-
      sorbent assay

el·lip·to·cy·ta·ry

el·lip·to·cyte

el·lip·to·cy·to·sis
   hemolytic e.
   hereditary e.

el·lip·to·cy·tot·ic

El·li·son
    Zollinger-E. syndrome

El·spar

El·trox·in

el·u·ate
    plasma barium citrate e.
    plasma barium sulfate e.

elu·tri·a·tion
    counterflow centrifugal e.

EMA
    etoposide, mitoxantrone,
        and cytarabine

EMA-CO
    etoposide, methotrexate,
        dactinomycin, cyclophos-
        phamide, and vincristine

EMAP
    endothelial cell macro-
        phage activating poly-
        peptide

Emb·den
    E.-Meyerhof pathway

em·bo·lism
    air e.

em·bo·lus *pl.* em·bo·li
    pulmonary e.

em·bry·o·ma
    e. of kidney

EM2 (myeloid) cell line

EM3 (myeloid) cell line

Em·cyt

em·e·sis
    cisplatin-induced e.

em·e·tine

em·e·to·gen·ic

em·i·gra·tion

EMIT
    enzyme-multiplied immu-
        noassay technique

en·am·elo·blas·to·ma

en·cap·su·lat·ed

en·cap·su·la·tion
    lysosomal e.

en·ceph·a·loid

en·ceph·a·lo·ma

en·chon·dro·sar·co·ma

en·do·car·di·tis
    thrombotic e.

en·do·cy·to·sis

en·do·derm

en·do·der·mal

en·do·glo·bar

en·do·glob·u·lar

en·do·gly·co·si·dase

en·do·me·tri·oid

en·do·me·tri·um *pl.* en·do·
    me·tria

en·do·myo·car·di·um

en·do·per·ox·ide
    platelet derived e.

en·do·sal·pin·go·ma

en·dos·co·py

en·do·sep·sis

en·dos·te·o·ma

en·dos·to·ma

en·do·the·lin

en·do·the·lio·blas·to·ma

en·do·the·lio·cyte

en·do·the·li·o·ma
    e. angiomatosum
    e. capitis

en·do·the·li·o·ma *(continued)*
    e. cutis
    diffuse e.
    dural e.
    perithelial e.

en·do·the·li·o·ma·to·sis

en·do·the·lio·sar·co·ma

en·do·the·li·um *pl.* en·do·the·lia

en·do·tox·e·mia

en·do·tox·in

en·do·tox·in·emia

En·drate

En·dur-Ac·in

en·e·ma *pl.* en·e·mas, e·nem·a·ta
    air-contrast barium e.
    barium e.
    double-contrast barium e.
    single-contrast barium e.

en·er·gy
    beam e.

en·globe

en·graft·ment
    myeloid e.

en·gulf·ment

en·hance·ment
    contrast e.

en·iso·prost

eno·lase
    neuron-specific e.

en·rich·ment
    stem cell e.

ENU
    N-ethyl-*N*-nitrosourea

enu·cle·a·tion

En·u·lose

en·zyme
    erythrocyte e.
    glycolytic e.
    liver e.
    PGO e's
    restriction e.

EORTC
    European Organization for Research on the Treatment of Cancer

eo·sin
    e. B
    e. Y

eo·sin·o·cyte

eo·sin·o·pe·nia

eo·sin·o·phil
    bone marrow e.

eo·sin·o·phile

eo·sin·o·phil·ia

eo·sin·o·phil·ic

eo·sin·o·phi·lo·sis

eo·sin·o·philo·tac·tic

eo·sin·oph·i·lous

eo·sin·o·tac·tic

EP
    erythrocyte protoporphyrin test
    etoposide and cisplatin

epen·dy·mo·blas·to·ma

epen·dy·mo·cy·to·ma

epen·dy·mo·ma

EPI
    extrinsic pathway inhibitor

ep·i·car·cin·o·gen

epi·der·mal

epi·der·mis *pl.* epi·der·mi·des

epi·der·moid

epi·der·moi·do·ma

epi·dox·o·ru·bi·cin

epi·ge·net·ic

epi·neph·rine

epi·neph·rin·emia

epi·podo·phyl·lo·tox·in

epi·ru·bi·cin

ep·i·stax·is

ep·i·the·li·o·ma
    e. adamantinum
    basal cell e.
    chorionic e.
    columnar e., cylindrical
    diffuse e.
    glandular e.
    malignant e.

ep·i·the·li·o·ma·to·sis

ep·i·the·li·o·ma·tous

ep·i·the·li·um *pl.* ep·i·the·
    lia
    glandular e.
    ovarian surface e.

ep·i·tope

ep·i·type

EPO
    erythropoietin

ep·o·pro·sten·ol

EPR-1
    effector cell protease re-
        ceptor-1

ep·si·lon-ami·no·ca·pro·ic
    acid

Ep·stein
    E.-Barr nuclear antigen
    E.-Barr virus

ER
    estrogen receptors

ERD
    extrapolated response dose

Er·gam·i·sol

er·go·cal·cif·er·ol

er·go·no·vine

Er·go·trate

er·i·o·nite

E-ro·sette

er·win·ia 1-as·par·a·gin·ase

Er·y·sip·elo·thrix
    E. rhusiopathiae

er·y·the·ma
    necrolytic migratory e.

er·y·thre·mia

eryth·ro·blast
    acidophilic e.
    basophilic e.
    early e.
    eosinophilic e.
    intermediate e.
    late e.
    orthochromatic e.
    oxyphilic e.
    polychromatic e.

eryth·ro·blas·te·mia

eryth·ro·blas·tic

eryth·ro·blas·to·ma

eryth·ro·blas·to·ma·to·sis

eryth·ro·blas·to·pe·nia
    idiopathic e.
    transient e. of childhood

eryth·ro·blas·to·sis
    e. fetalis

eryth·ro·blas·tot·ic

eryth·ro·ca·tal·y·sis

er·y·throc·la·sis

eryth·ro·clast

eryth·ro·clas·tic

eryth·ro·cy·ta·phe·re·sis

eryth·ro·cyte
    immature e.
    normochromic e.
    nucleated e.
    orthochromatic e.
    polychromatic e.
    polychromatophilic e.
    sickled e.
    TN e.

eryth·ro·cyt·ic

eryth·ro·cy·to·blast

eryth·ro·cy·tol·y·sin

eryth·ro·cy·tol·y·sis

eryth·ro·cy·tom·e·ter

eryth·ro·cy·tom·e·try

eryth·ro·cy·to-op·so·nin

eryth·ro·cy·to·pe·nia

eryth·ro·cy·toph·a·gous

eryth·ro·cy·toph·a·gy

eryth·ro·cy·to·poi·e·sis

eryth·ro·cy·tor·rhex·is

eryth·ro·cy·tos·chi·sis

eryth·ro·cy·to·sis
    leukemic e.
    paraneoplastic e.
    stress e.

eryth·ro·de·gen·er·a·tive

eryth·ro·gen·e·sis
    e. imperfecta

eryth·ro·gen·ic

er·y·throid

eryth·ro·ka·tal·y·sis

eryth·ro·ki·net·ics

eryth·ro·leu·ke·mia
    acute e.
    Friend murine e. (F-MEL)
    human e. (HEL)

eryth·ro·leu·ko·throm·bo·cy·the·mia

er·y·throl·y·sin

er·y·throl·y·sis

er·y·throm·e·ter

er·y·throm·e·try

eryth·ro·my·cin

er·y·thron

eryth·ro·neo·cy·to·sis

eryth·ro·no·clas·tic

eryth·ro·pe·nia

eryth·ro·phage

eryth·ro·pha·gia

eryth·ro·phago·cyt·ic

eryth·ro·phago·cy·to·sis

er·y·throph·a·gous

eryth·ro·pla·sia
    e. of Queyrat

eryth·ro·plas·tid

eryth·ro·poi·e·sis
    extramedullary e.
    ineffective e.

eryth·ro·poi·et·ic

eryth·ro·poi·e·tin

eryth·ror·rhex·is

eryth·ro·sed·i·men·ta·tion

er·y·thro·sis

eryth·ro·sta·sis

Esch·e·rich·ia
    E. coli

Esh
     E. sarcoma virus

ESMO
     European Society for Medical Oncology

esoph·a·gec·to·my

esoph·a·go·gas·trec·to·my

esoph·a·go·gas·trot·o·my

esoph·a·gus
     Barrett's e.

eso·ru·bi·cin

es·sen·tial

es·ter
     phorbol e.

es·ter·ase

es·the·sio·neu·ro·blas·to·ma

es·the·sio·neu·ro·cy·to·ma

es·the·sio·neu·ro·epi·the·li·o·ma

es·the·sio·neu·ro·ma

Es·ti·nyl

es·tra·di·ol
     e. valerate

Es·tra·di·ol L.A.

Es·tra-L

es·tra·mus·tine

Es·tra·tab

Es·tra·val

es·tro·gen
     conjugated e's
     esterified e's

es·tro·gen·ic

es·tro·gen-re·cep·tor pos·i·tive

Es·tro·ject-2

es·trone

Es·tro·nol

es·tro·phil·in

ETA
     etanidazole

Eta
     etanidazole

et·a·ni·da·zole

eth·a·cryn·ic acid

eth·a·nol

ether
     bis(chlormethyl) e.
     chloromethyl methyl e.

eth·i·nyl es·tra·di·ol

ethi·o·fos

etho·glu·cid

eth·y·lene di·bro·mide

eth·y·lene di·ox·ide

eth·yl·en·i·mine

N-eth·yl-*N*-ni·tro·so·urea

Eth·y·ol

eti·dro·nate

etio·cho·lan·o·lone

ETOP
     etoposide

Etop
     etoposide

eto·po·side

Eu·flex

eu·glo·bin

eu·gly·ce·mia

eu·gly·ce·mic

Eu·lex·in

Eu·ro·pe·an Or·ga·ni·za·tion for Re·search on the Treat·ment of Can·cer

Eu·ro·pe·an So·ci·e·ty for Med·i·cal On·col·o·gy

Eu·throid

EVA
    etoposide, vincristine, dox-
        orubicin

EVAC
    etoposide, vincristine, dox-
        orubicin, and cyclophos-
        phamide

Ev·ans
    E. blue
    E. staging (for neuroblas-
        toma)
    E. syndrome

EVAP
    etoposide, vinblastine, cy-
        tarabine, and cisplatin

Ev·er·one

E-Vis·ta

Ewald
    E's node

Ew·ing
    E's sarcoma
    E's tumor

ex·am·i·na·tion
    digital e.
    digital rectal e.

ex·change
    plasma e.

ex·ci·sion
    full-thickness local e.
    wide e.

ex·e·mia

ex·en·ter·a·tion
    pelvic e.

ex·fo·li·a·tive

exo·phyt·ic

ex·os·to·sis
    e. cartilaginea
    cartilaginous exostoses
    osteocartilaginous e.

exo·the·li·o·ma

exo·tox·in
    Pseudomonas e.

ex·pan·der
    plasma volume e.

ex·pan·sile

ex·pan·sion
    clonal e.

ex·po·sure
    occupational e.
    workplace e.

ex·pres·sion
    gene e.
    mixed-lineage e.

ex·san·gui·no·trans·fu·sion

ex·ten·der
    artificial plasma e.

ex·ten·sion
    extrascleral e.
    lymphatic e.
    tumor e.

ex·tra·cel·lu·lar

ex·tra·cor·pus·cu·lar

ex·tract
    Serratia marcescens e.

ex·tra·he·pat·ic

ex·tra·lym·phat·ic

ex·tra·no·dal

ex·tra·oc·u·lar

ex·tra·os·se·ous

Fab
    fragment, antigen-binding

F(ab)₂
    the fragment obtained by
    pepsin cleavage of the
    IgG molecule

F(ab')₂
    symbol for a fragment of
    an immunoglobulin G
    molecule

FAB (French-American-
    British) clas·si·fi·ca·tion
    (for acute lymphoblastic and
    myelogenous leukemias)

Fa·ber
    F's syndrome

fa·bism

Fa·bri·ci·us
    bursa of F.

Fa·bry
    F's syndrome

FAC
    5-fluorouracil, doxorubicin,
    and cyclophosphamide

Facb
    fragment, antigen- and
    complement-binding

FACP
    fluorouracil, doxorubicin,
    cyclophosphamide, and
    cisplatin

FACS
    fluorescence-activated cell
    sorter

fac·tor
    Factor I
    Factor II
    Factor III
    Factor IV

fac·tor (continued)
    Factor V
    Factor VI
    Factor VII
    Factor VIII
    Factor IX
    Factor X
    Factor XI
    Factor XII
    Factor XIII
    f. A
    accelerator f.
    acidified serum lysis f.
    activation f.
    ADP-sensitive f.
    antigen-specific T-cell
      helper f.
    antigen-specific T-cell sup-
      pressor f.
    antihemophilic f.
    antihemophilic f. A
    antihemophilic f. B
    antihemophilic f. C
    AP1 f.
    asialo-von Willebrand f.
    autocrine f.
    autocrine growth f.
    f. B
    basophil chemotactic f.
      (BCF)
    B cell differentiation f's
      (BCDF)
    B cell growth f's (BCGF)
    B cell stimulatory f.
    B cell stimulatory f. 1
    B cell stimulatory f. 2
    blastogenic f. (BF)
    B-lymphocyte stimulatory
      f's (BSF)
    cell migration f.
    Chapel Hill IX f.
    Christmas f.
    clonal inhibitory f.
    cloning inhibitory f.

fac·tor *(continued)*

coagulant f. VIII (VIIIc)
coagulation f.'s
colony-stimulating f. (CSF)
conglutinogen activating f. (KAF)
contact f.
D-f.
f. D
decarboxy f. IX
decay-accelerating f.
decay-activating f. (DAF)
Deventer IX f.
eosinophil chemotactic f. (ECF)
eosinophil chemotactic f. of anaphylaxis (ECF-A)
eosinophil differentiation f. (EDF)
erythrocyte-stimulating f.
erythroid colony stimulating f. (E-CSF)
erythropoietic stimulating f. (ESF)
fibrin stabilizing f.
fibroblast growth f.
Fitzgerald f.
Fitzgerald-Williams-Flaujeac f.
Fleaujeac f.
Fletcher f.
Friuli f. X
GATA transcription f.
glass f.
granulocyte colony stimulating f.
granulocyte-macrophage colony stimulating f.
granulocyte macrophage-colony stimulating f., recombinant E (rGM-CSF)
growth f.
growth inhibitory f's
f. H
Hageman f. (HF)
hematopoietic growth f's
heparin-binding fibroblast growth f.

fac·tor *(continued)*

high-molecular-weight neutrophil chemotactic f. (HMW-NCF)
histamine releasing f.
host-related f.
human colony-stimulating f.
hybridoma/plasmacytoma growth f.
hydrazine-sensitive f. (HSF)
immunoglobulin-binding f. (IBF)
interferon response f.
interferon response f. 1
interferon response f. 2
labile f.
Laki-Lorand f.
leukemia inhibitory f. (LIF)
leukocyte inhibitory f. (LIF)
lymphocyte activating f.
lymphocyte blastogenic f. (BF)
lymphocyte mitogenic f. (LMF)
lymphocyte transforming f. (LTF)
macrophage-activating f. (MAF)
macrophage chemotactic f. (MCF)
macrophage colony-stimulating f. (M-CSF)
macrophage-derived growth f.
macrophage growth f. (MGF)
macrophage inhibitory f. (MIF)
mast cell f.
megakaryocytic colony stimulating f.
migration inhibiting f. (MIF)
mitogenic f.

fac·tor *(continued)*
    monoclonal f. IX
    multicolony-stimulating f. (multi-CSF)
    multilineage colony-stimulating f.
    natural killer cell stimulatory f.
    natural killer cytotoxic f.
    neutrophil chemotactic f. (NCF)
    neutrophil immobilizing f.
    nuclear f.
    f. P
    Passovoy f.
    P-cell growth f.
    P40 growth f.
    platelet f's
    platelet f. 1
    platelet f. 2
    platelet f. 3
    platelet f. 4
    platelet activating f. (PAF)
    platelet-derived growth f.
    proconvertin stable f.
    proliferation inhibitory f. (PIF)
    prothrombokinase f.
    Prower f.
    P40 T-cell growth f.
    purified F. VIII
    recruitment f.
    Reid f.
    Rh f.
    Rhesus f.
    specific macrophage arming f. (SMAF)
    stable f.
    stem cell f.
    Stuart f.
    Stuart-Prower f.
    TATA f.
    T-cell growth f.
    T cell replacing f.
    tissue f.
    transcription f.
    transfer f. (TF)
    transforming growth f.

fac·tor *(continued)*
    transforming growth f. α
    transforming growth factor alpha
    transforming growth f. β
    transforming growth f. β₁
    transforming growth f. beta
    tumor-angiogenesis f.
    tumor autocrine mobility f.
    tumor necrosis f. (TNF)
    tumor necrosis f. α
    tumor necrosis f. β
    vitamin K–dependent f.
    von Willebrand's f.
    Washington f.
    Willebrand's blood coagulation f.
    Williams f.
    f. X *Friuli*
    Zutphen IX f.

Fac·tor VIIIag
    Factor VIII–related antigen

Fah·rae·us
    F. method
    F.-Lindqvist effect

fail·ure
    acute renal f.
    bone marrow f.

fal·ca·di·na

Falls
    Rundles-F. syndrome

FAM
    5-fluorouracil, doxorubicin, and mitomycin

FAMe
    5-fluorouracil, doxorubicin, and semustine

fam·i·ly
    SIG (small inducible gene) f.

FAMMM (familial atypical multiple mole melanoma) syndrome

Fan·co·ni
    F's anemia
    F's disease
    F's pancytopenia
    F's pancytopenia syndrome
    F. syndrome

FAP
    familial adenomatous polyposis
    5-fluorouracil, doxorubicin, and cisplatin

Farre
    F's tubercle

fas·ci·itis
    diffuse f.
    nodular f.
    pseudosarcomatous f.

FAT
    5-fluorouracil, doxorubicin, and trazinate

fat
    dietary f.

fat·ty ac·id

fa·vism

Fc
    fragment, crystallizable

Fc'
    a fragment produced by papain digestion of the IgG molecule

FCC
    fibrocystic changes
    follicular center cells

Fd
    the heavy chain portion of the Fab fragment

FDC-P1 (myeloid) cell line

FEC
    fluorouracil, cyclophosphamide, and epirubicin

fem·i·ni·za·tion

Fem·i·none

Fem·o·gen For·te

Fem·o·gex

fe·mur pl. fem·o·ra

Fendt
    Spiegler-F. sarcoid

FEP
    5-fluorouracil, epirubicin, and cisplatin

Fer·ra·ta
    F's cell

fer·ri·tin
    serum f.

fer·ro·cy·a·nide
    acid f.

fer·ro·ki·net·ic

fer·ro·ki·net·ics

fe·ver
    blackwater f.
    familial Mediterranean f.
    Pel-Ebstein f.

FFR
    freedom from relapse

FGF
    fibroblast growth factor

fi·ber
    dietary f.
    Rosenthal's f's

fi·bril·lary

fi·brin
    f. cross-linking
    stroma f.

fi·brin·ase

fi·bri·no·cel·lu·lar

fi·brin·o·gen
 f. *Alba/Geneva*
 f. *Amsterdam*
 f. *Baltimore*
 f. *Bern II*
 f. *Bethesda I*
 f. *Bethesda II*
 f. *Bethesda III*
 f. *Bicêtre*
 f. *Buenos Aires*
 f. *Caracas*
 f. *Chapel Hill I*
 f. *Charlottesville*
 f. *Cleveland I*
 f. *Cleveland II*
 f. *Copenhagen*
 f. *Detroit*
 f. *Giessen I*
 f. *Giessen II*
 f. *Giessen III*
 f. *Hanover*
 f. *Iowa City*
 f. *Istanbul I*
 f. *Leuven*
 f. *Lille*
 f. *London*
 f. *Los Angeles*
 f. *Louisville*
 f. *Manchester*
 f. *Manila*
 f. *Marburg*
 f. *Metz*
 f. *Mexico City*
 f. *Montreal I*
 f. *Montreal II*
 f. *Munich I*
 f. *Nancy*
 f. *New Albany*
 f. *New Orleans*
 f. *New York*
 f. *Oklahoma City*
 f. *Oslo I*
 f. *Oslo II*
 f. *Paris I*
 f. *Paris II*
 f. *Paris III*
 f. *Parma*
 f. *Parnham*

fi·brin·o·gen *(continued)*
 f. *Petroskey*
 f. *Philadelphia*
 f. *Pontoise*
 f. *Quebec I*
 f. *Quebec II*
 f. *Rouen*
 f. *Schwartzach*
 f. *Seattle*
 f. *Spokane*
 f. *St. Louis*
 f. *Sydney I*
 f. *Sydney II*
 f. *Tokyo*
 f. *Troyes*
 f. *Valencia*
 f. *Vancouver*
 f. *Vienna*
 f. *White Marsh*
 f. *Wiesbaden*
 f. *Zurich I*
 f. *Zurich II*

fi·brin·og·en·ase

fi·brin·o·gen·emia

fi·bri·no·gen·e·sis

fi·bri·no·gen·ic

fi·bri·no·ge·nol·y·sis

fi·bri·no·geno·lyt·ic

fi·brin·o·geno·pe·nia

fi·brin·o·geno·pe·nic

fi·bri·nog·e·nous

fi·bri·no·ki·nase

fi·bri·no·li·gase

fi·bri·nol·y·sis

fi·bri·no·lyt·ic

fi·bri·no·nec·tin

fi·bri·no·pe·nia

fi·bri·no·pep·tide
 f. A
 f. B

fi·bri·no·plate·let

fi·brin·ous

fil·gras·tim

fi·brin-spe·cif·ic

fi·bro·ad·e·no·ma

fi·bro·an·gi·o·ma

fi·bro·blast

fi·bro·blas·to·ma

fi·bro·car·ci·no·ma

fi·bro·chon·dro·ma

fi·bro·cyst

fi·bro·cys·to·ma

fi·bro·en·chon·dro·ma

fi·bro·ep·i·the·li·o·ma
  premalignant f.

fi·bro·gam·min

fi·bro·ge·nol·y·sis

fi·bro·gli·o·ma

fi·broid

fi·bro·la·mel·lar

fi·bro·li·po·ma

fi·bro·li·po·ma·tous

fi·bro·ma
  ameloblastic f.
  f. cavernosum
  chondromyxoid f.
  f. cutis
  cystic f.
  desmoplastic f.
  f. durum
  hard f.
  intracanalicular f.
  juvenile aponeurotic f.
  f. mucinosum
  f. myxomatodes
  ossifying f.
  ossifying f. of bone

fi·bro·ma *(continued)*
  osteogenic f.
  f. sarcomatosum
  telangiectatic f.

fi·bro·ma·to·gen·ic

fi·bro·ma·toid

fi·bro·ma·to·sis

fi·bro·ma·tous

fi·bro·mec·to·my

fi·bro·myx·o·ma

fi·bro·myx·o·sar·co·ma

fi·bro·nec·tin

fi·bro-os·te·o·ma

fi·bro·pap·il·lo·ma

fi·bro·sar·co·ma
  f. of bone
  primary f.

fi·bro·sis
  hyaline f.
  pulmonary f.

Fi·che·ra
  F's method

Fi·coll

field
  anterior-posterior f.
  lateral f.
  mantle f.
  posterior-anterior f.
  preauricular f.
  spade f.
  subdiaphragmatic f.
  supradiaphragmatic f.
  tangential f.
  vertex f.
  Waldeyer f.

FIGO
  International Federation
    of Gynecology and Ob-
    stetrics

FIGO stag·ing (for ovarian cancer)

fig·ure
    mitotic f's

fil·a·min

fi·li·pod

film
    localization f.
    plain f.

fi·lo·po·dia

fil·tra·tion
    microporous membrane f.

fin·ger·print·ing
    DNA f.

first mes·sen·ger

Fish·er
    F. blood group

Fiske & Sub·ba·Row reducer

Fitz·ger·ald
    F. factor
    F. trait
    F.-Williams-Flaujeac factor

fix·a·tion
    complement f.
    f. of complement

FJP
    familial juvenile polyposis

Flau·jeac
    Fitzgerald-Williams-F. factor
    F. factor
    F. trait

fla·vone ace·tic acid

Flet·cher
    F. factor
    F. trait

floc·cu·la·tion

flow
    shear f.

flox·uri·dine

flu·car·a·bine

flu·con·a·zole

fluc·tu·ant

flu·dar·a·bine
    f. monophosphate
    f. phosphate

flu·de·oxy·glu·cose F 18

flu·id
    Callison's f.
    cerebrospinal f. (CSF)
    Ecker's f.
    Piazza's f.
    Rees and Ecker diluting f.
    synovial f.
    Toison's f.

flu·o·ro-AMP

flu·o·ro·cyte

[^{18}F] flu·o·ro·de·oxy·glu·cose

flu·o·ro·de·oxy·uri·dine mono·phos·phate

flu·o·ro·do·pan

flu·o·ro·im·mu·no·as·say

flu·o·ro·meth·o·lone

flu·o·ro·py·rim·i·dine

flu·o·ro·ura·cil

5-flu·o·ro·ura·cil

Flu·o·sol

flu·ox·y·mes·ter·one

flu·ro·ci·ta·bine

5-flu·ro-2-de·oxy·uri·dine

flush
    carcinoid f.

flush·ing
  idiopathic f.

flu·ta·mide

flux·uri·dine

F-MACHOP
  fluorouracil, methotrexate,
  doxorubicin, cytarabine,
  cyclophosphamide, vin-
  cristine, and prednisone

F-MEL
  Friend murine erythroleukemia

FOBT
  fecal occult blood test

fo·late

fold
  aryepiglottic f.

Fo·lex

fol·ic acid

Fo·lin
  F. and Wu's method

fol·li·cle
  colonic lymphoid f.

fol·lic·u·lo·ma
  f. lipidique

Fo·nio
  F's solution

Fon·ta·na
  F.-Masson stain

foot·print·ing
  DNAase f.

force
  flow/shear f.

form
  α f.
  band f's
  juvenile f.
  young f.

for·mal·de·hyde

for·ma·lin

for·ma·tion
  antibody f.
  palisade f.
  rouleaux f.

for·mu·la *pl.* for·mu·lae, for·
mu·las
  Arneth's f.

for·myl-me·thi·o·nyl-leu·cyl-
  phen·yl·al·a·nine

for·sko·lin

fos·fo·my·cin

fos gene

Foy·gen Aq·ue·ous

FPC
  familial polyposis coli

FR
  family report

frac·tion
  Blömback f. I-0
  Cohn f. I
  plasma f's
  S-phase f.

frac·tion·a·tion
  accelerated f.
  classical f.
  conventional f.
  dose f.

frac·ture
  pathologic f.

fra·gil·i·ty
  f. of blood
  erythrocyte f.
  mechanical f.
  osmotic f.

fra·gilo·cyte

fra·gilo·cy·to·sis

frag·ment
  Eco Ri f.
  Fab f.

frag·ment *(continued)*
    F(ab')$_2$ f.
    Fc f.
    restriction f.

frame·shift

Frank·lin
    F's disease

Fran·me·ni
    Li-F. syndrome

freck·le
    melanotic f. of Hutchinson

fre·quen·cy
    HLA f.

Freund
    F's adjuvant

Friend
    F. murine erythroleuke-
        mia (F-MEL)
    F. virus

Friu·li
    F. factor X

Frosst·image MAA

Frosst·image Sul·fur Col·loid

fruc·tos·emia

fruc·tose-2-phos·phate

FS
    Felty's syndrome

FSF
    fibrin-stabilizing factor

FT-207

FTLE
    full-thickness local exci-
        sion

Ftor·a·fur

FTS-Zn
    thymulin

FU
    fluorouracil

5-FU
    5-fluorouracil

Fu
    fluorouracil

5-Fu
    5-fluorouracil

FUDR
    fluorodeoxyuridine

Fu·ji·na·mi
    F. sarcoma virus

ful·gu·ra·tion

Ful·thorpe
    Oakley-F. technique
    Oakley-F. test

5-Fu + Lv
    5-fluorouracil and leucovo-
        rin

fu·ma·rate
    ferrous f.

func·tion
    platelet f.

fu·ro·sem·ide

fu·si·dic

FV
    Friend virus

GAA→TAA mu·ta·tion

gad·o·lin·i·um
    g. DTPA

gad·o·pen·te·tate di·me·glu·mine

Gais·böck
    G's disease
    G's syndrome

gal·ac·te·mia

ga·lac·ti·tol

β-ga·lac·to·si·dase

gall·blad·der

gal·li·um
    g. citrate radionuclide
    g. nitrate

GalNAc (β1,3)-D-ga·lac·to·syl trans·fer·ase

GALT
    gut-associated lymphatic tissue

Ga·mi·mune N

gam·ma glob·u·lin

gam·ma·glob·u·li·nop·a·thy

gam·ma-glu·ta·myl cys·te·ine syn·the·tase

gam·ma-glu·ta·myl cys·te·ine syn·the·tase de·fi·cien·cy

gam·mop·a·thy
    benign monoclonal g.
    monoclonal g.
    monoclonal g. of undetermined significance (MGUS)

gan·ci·clo·vir

gan·gli·on *pl.* gan·glia, gan·gli·ons
    Troisier's g.

gan·glio·neu·ro·blas·to·ma

gan·glio·neu·ro·ma

gan·glio·side

Gan·ite

GAP ki·nase

Gard·ner
    G's syndrome

gar·goyl·ism

gas
    mustard g.

Gas·ser
    G's syndrome

gas·trec·to·my

gas·tric

gas·tri·no·ma

Gas·tro·in·tes·ti·nal Tu·mor Stu·dy Group

GATA tran·scrip·tion fac·tor

gat·ing
    B cell g.

Gau·cher
    G's disease

G-band·ing

GBM
    glioblastoma multiforme

GCP
    granulocyte chemotactic protein

G-CSF
    granulocyte colony stimulating factor

Gd
    gadolinium

Gd DTPA
    gadolinium DTPA

gel
    g. filtration

Gell
    G. and Coombs classifica-
      tion

gel·sol·in

Gel·u·sil

gem·fib·ro·zil

ge·mis·to·cyte

ge·mis·to·cyt·ic

gene
    abl g.
    axl g.
    bcl-1 g.
    bcl-2 g.
    bcr g.
    bcr-abl fusion g.
    beta-Montreal g.
    B-*myb* g.
    calcitonin g.
    DNA virus transforming
      g.
    egr-1 g.
    g. expression
    fos g.
    globin g.
    H (histocompatibility) g.
    H-2K^b g.
    Ha-*ras* g.
    hck g.
    histocompatibility g.
    homeobox g.
    HSP70 g.
    In(Lu) g.
    jun g.
    MDR (multidrug resis-
      tance) g.
    MDR1 g.
    mol g.
    multidrug resistance g.

gene *(continued)*
    nef g.
    neo g.
    NF-*jun* g.
    N-*myc* g.
    P53 tumor suppressor g.
    pol g.
    rev g.
    rex g.
    small inducible g.
    suppressor g.
    tumor necrosis factor-β g.
    tumor suppressor g.
    vif g.

Gen·er·lac

ge·net·ics
    molecular g.

Gen·gou
    Bordet-G. phenomenon
    G. phenomenon

Gen-K

geno·tox·ic

geno·type

geno·typ·ic

ger·mi·no·ma

Ges·ter·ol L.A.

GFAP
    glial fibrillary acidic pro-
      tein

GFCL
    giant follicular cell lym-
      phoma

ghost
    red cell g.

Gied·i·on
    Langer-G. syndrome

Giem·sa
    G. banding
    G. stain
    Wright-G. stain

Gil·bert
    G's disease

GITSG
Gastrointestinal Tumor
Study Group

G-ki·nase

G.K. var·i·ant

gland
adrenal g.
Bartholin's g.
parathyroid g's
parotid g.
salivary g's
thyroid g.
Virchow's g.

G pro·tein

Glanz·mann
G's disease
G's thrombasthenia

glio·blas·to·ma
g. multiforme

glio·cy·to·ma

gli·o·ma
astrocytic g.
brainstem g.
ependymal g.
ganglionic g.
low-grade astrocytic g.
midbrain g.
mixed g.
nasal g.
optic g.
peripheral g.
postradiation g.
g. sarcomatosum
spinal cord g.
telangiectatic g.

gli·o·ma·tous

glio·neu·ro·ma

glio·sar·co·ma

glo·bin
α g.
α₂ g.
β g.
Γ d.

glo·bin (continued)
γ g.

glo·bi·nom·e·ter

glob·u·lin
AC g.
accelerator g.
antihemophilic g. (AHG)
antilymphocyte g. (ALG)
antithymocyte g. (ATG)
gamma g's
hepatitis B immune g.

glo·mus pl. glo·me·ra
g. jugulare

glot·tis pl. glot·ti·des

glu·ca·gon

glu·ca·gon·o·ma

glu·ce·mia

glu·co·cer·e·bro·si·dase

glu·co·cor·ti·coid

glu·co·he·mia

glu·co·nate
ferrous g.

glu·cose

glu·cose-6-phos·phate

glu·cose-6-phos·phate de·hy·dro·gen·ase (G6PD)

glu·cose-6-phos·phate de·hy·dro·gen·ase (G6PD) deficiency

glu·cose-6-phos·phate isom·er·ase

glu·cose-6-phos·phate isom·er·ase de·fi·cien·cy

β-glu·co·si·dase

Glu-plas·min·o·gen

glu·ta·mate de·hy·dro·gen·ase

glu·ta·mine

glu·ta·ral·de·hyde

glu·ta·thi·one

glu·ta·thi·one per·ox·i·dase

glu·ta·thi·one per·ox·i·dase
  de·fi·cien·cy

glu·ta·thi·one re·duc·tase
  (NAD(P)H)

glu·ta·thi·one re·duc·tase
  de·fi·cien·cy

glu·ta·thi·one syn·the·tase

glu·ta·thi·one syn·the·tase
  de·fi·cien·cy

glu·ta·thi·one-*S*-trans·fer·
  ase

glu·ta·thi·on·emia

glu·teth·i·mide

gly·can·ase

gly·ce·mia

glyc·er·ol·ize

glyc·ero·phos·phate

gly·cine

gly·co·cal·i·cin

gly·co·he·mia

gly·co·he·mo·glo·bin

gly·col·y·sis

gly·co·lyt·ic

gly·co·phor·in
  g. A
  α g.
  g. B
  β₂-g. I
  δ g.
  MiV g.
  MiV(J.L.) g.
  Stᵃ g.

gly·co·pro·tein
  g. Ia
  g. Ib
  g. Ib/IX
  g. Ic
  g. Ic/IIa
  g. IIa
  g. IIb
  g. IIb/IIIa
  g. IIIa
  g. IV
  g. V
  g. IX
  glycine-rich β g. (GBG)
  tumor-associated g.

gly·cos·ami·no·gly·can

gly·co·se·mia

gly·co·syl·a·tion

glyc·yl·tryp·to·phan

GM-CSF
  granulocyte-macrophage
  colony-stimulating factor

GMP
  guanosine monophosphate

GMP-140
  granule membrane protein

GOG
  Gynecologic Oncology
  Group

goi·ter

gold
  radioactive g.

Gold·ie
  G.-Coldman hypothesis

gom·pert·zi·an cell ki·net·ics

gom·pert·zi·an growth

gon·a·do·blas·to·ma

gon·a·do·tro·pin
  human chorionic g. (hCG)

Good
    G's syndrome

Good·pas·ture
    G's syndrome

Gor·don
    G's biological test
    G's elementary body

Gor·lin
    G. syndrome

go·se·rel·in

Gow·er
    G. hemoglobin

Gow·ers
    G. solution

GP
    glycoprotein

gp
    glycoprotein

G6PD
    glucose-6-phosphate dehy-
      drogenase

G-6-PD de·fi·cien·cy

grade
    Broder's g.
    histological g.

grad·ing
    toxicity g.

Gras·beck
    Imerslund-G. syndrome

graft
    allogeneic g.
    allogenic g.
    autochthonous g.
    autogenous g.
    autologous g.
    autoplastic g.
    heterologous g.
    heteroplastic g.
    homologous g.
    homoplastic g.
    isogeneic g.

graft *(continued)*
    isologous g.
    isoplastic g.
    marrow g.
    syngeneic g.

graft-ver·sus-host

graft-ver·sus-leu·ke·mia

gran·i·se·tron

gran·u·la·tion
    Reilly g's
    toxic g.

gran·ule
    alpha g's
    azur g.
    azurophil g.
    azurophilic g.
    basophil g's
    "bull's eye" g.
    delta g's
    dense g.
    elementary g's
    hyperchromatin g.
    kappa g.
    lysosome g.
    platelet g.
    primary g.

gran·u·lo·blast

gran·u·lo·cyte
    band-form g.
    segmented g.

gran·u·lo·cyt·ic

gran·u·lo·cy·top·a·thy

gran·u·lo·cy·to·pe·nia

gran·u·lo·cy·to·poi·e·sis

gran·u·lo·cy·to·poi·et·ic

gran·u·lo·cy·to·sis

gran·u·lo·ma *pl.* gran·u·lo·
mas, gran·u·lo·ma·ta
    Hodgkin's g.
    reticulohistiocytic g.

gran·u·lo·ma·to·sis
    lymphomatoid g.
    malignant g.

gran·u·lo·mere

gran·u·lo·pe·nia

gran·u·lo·poi·e·sis

gran·u·lo·poi·et·ic

gran·u·lo·poi·e·tin

Grase·by pump

Graves
    G. disease

Gra·witz
    G's tumors

gray

green
    diazin g. S
    Janus g. B
    light g. S F yellowish
    union g. B

Gri·scel·li
    G. syndrome

gris·eo·ful·vin

Gro·shong
    G. catheter
    G. port

group
    blood g.
    Carcinogen Assessment G.

growth
    gompertzian g.

Grün·wald
    May-G. stain
    Gardner syndrome

GS

GSH
    glutathione

GST
    glutathione-S-transferase

guai·fen·e·sin

guan·i·din·emia

Gué·rin
    bacille Calmette-G.
    Calmette-G. bacillus
      (BCG)

Gun Hill
    hemoglobin G.H.

Gy
    gray

gy·nan·dro·blas·to·ma

Gyne·co·log·ic On·col·o·gy
  Group

Gyn·o·gen

H

H
doxorubicin (hydroxydau-
norubicin)

Ha·ber
H.-Weiss reaction

haem

Hae·moph·i·lus
H. ducreyi
H. influenzae

Hag·e·man
H. factor
H. trait

HAI
hepatic artery infusion

HAI (hemagglutination
inhibition) as·say

HAI (hemagglutination
inhibition) test

half-time
plasma iron clearance h.

ha·lom·e·ter

ha·lom·e·try

Hal·o·tes·tin

Ham
H. test

HAMA
human antimouse anti-
body

ham·ar·to·blas·to·ma

ham·ar·to·ma
angiomatous lymphoid h.
fetal renal h.
fibrous h. of infancy
renal h.

ham·ar·to·ma·to·sis

ham·ar·to·ma·tous

Ham·burg·er
H. interchange
H. phenomenon

Hank
H's balanced salt solution

hap·loid

hap·lo·type
Senegal h.

Haps·burg
disease of the H's

hap·ten

hap·ten·ic

hap·to·glo·bin

Ha-*ras* gene

Hare
H's syndrome

har·vest
marrow h.

har·vest·ing
bone marrow h.

Hash·i·mo·to
H's thyroiditis

Has·sell
H's corpuscle

Ha·yem
H's solution
H.-Widal syndrome

HBFG
heparin-binding fibroblast
growth factor

HBIG
hepatitis B immune globu-
lin

HC II
heparin cofactor II

H-CAm
   homing-associated adhe-
      sion molecule

H-CAP
   hexamethylmelamine, cy-
      clophosphamide, doxoru-
      bicin, and cisplatin

HCD-57 cell

hCG
   human chorionic gonado-
      tropin

β-hCG
   beta-human chorionic go-
      nadotropin

H (heavy) chain

hck gene

HCL
   hairy cell leukemia

HCRT
   high-resolution computed
      tomography

HD
   Hodgkin's disease

HD37-SAP im·mu·no·tox·in

HD39-SAP im·mu·no·tox·in

H&E
   hematoxylin and eosin
      (stain)

heat·ing
   tumor h.

Heck·a·thorn
   H's disease

Heg·glin
   May-H. anomaly

Heinz
   H. bodies
   H. body anemias
   H. body hemolytic anemia
   congenital H. body hemo-
      lytic anemia

HEL
   human erythroleukemia

HEM
   hexamethylmelamine, eto-
      poside, and methotrexate

He·ma·bate

hema·chrome

hema·cyte

hema·cy·tom·e·ter

hema·cy·tom·e·try

hem·ad·sor·bent

hem·ad·sorp·tion

hema·fa·cient

hem·ag·glu·ti·na·tion
   indirect h.
   passive h.

hem·ag·glu·ti·na·tive

hem·ag·glu·ti·nin
   cold h.
   warm h.

hem·a·nal·y·sis

hem·an·gio·amelo·blas·to·
   ma

hem·an·gio·blast

hem·an·gio·blas·to·ma

hem·an·gio·en·do·the·lio·
   blas·to·ma

hem·an·gio·en·do·the·li·o·
   ma
   benign h.
   epithelioid h.
   malignant h.

hem·an·gio·en·do·the·lio·
   sar·co·ma

hem·an·gi·o·ma
   ameloblastic h.
   h. cavernosum
   cavernous h.

hem·an·gio·peri·cy·to·ma

hem·an·gio·sar·co·ma

hema·phe·re·sis

hema·poi·e·sis

hema·poi·et·ic

hem·ar·thro·sis

He·ma-Tek

he·mat·ic

hem·a·tim·e·ter

hem·a·tim·e·try

hem·a·tin·emia

hem·a·tin·om·e·ter

hem·a·to·blast

hem·a·to·che·zia

he·ma·to·crit
    large vessel h.
    total body h.
    whole body h.
    Wintrobe h.

hem·a·to·cyte

hem·a·to·cy·to·blast

hem·a·to·cy·tol·y·sis

hem·a·to·cy·tom·e·ter

hem·a·to·cy·to·pe·nia

hem·a·to·gen·e·sis

hem·a·to·gen·ic

hem·a·tog·e·nous

hem·a·to·glo·bin

hem·a·to·gone

he·ma·to·his·tio·blast

hem·a·toid

hem·a·toid·in

hem·a·tol·o·gist

hem·a·tol·o·gy

hem·a·to·lymph·an·gi·o·ma

hem·a·tol·y·sis

hem·a·to·lyt·ic

hem·a·tom·e·ter

hem·a·tom·e·try

hem·a·to·pa·thol·o·gy

hem·a·to·pe·nia

hem·a·to·phage

hem·a·to·pha·gia

he·ma·to·phago·cyte

hem·a·toph·a·gous

hem·a·toph·a·gy

hem·a·to·phil·ia

hem·a·to·plas·tic

hem·a·to·poi·e·sis
    cyclic h.
    extramedullary h.

hem·a·to·poi·et·ic

hem·a·to·poi·e·tin

hem·a·to·por·phy·rin

hem·a·to·por·phy·rin·emia

hem·a·to·spec·tro·pho·tom·e·ter

hem·a·to·spec·tro·scope

hem·a·to·spec·tros·co·py

hem·a·to·spher·in·emia

hem·a·to·stat·ic

hem·a·to·tox·ic

hem·a·to·tox·i·co·sis

hem·a·to·trop·ic

hem·a·tox·ic

he·ma·tox·y·lin

hem·a·tu·ria

heme

He·med catheter

hem·en·do·the·li·o·ma

Heme·Se·lect

he·mic

he·min

hem·iso·ton·ic

he·mo·ag·glu·ti·na·tion

he·mo·ag·glu·ti·nin

he·mo·blast
    lymphoid h. of Pappen-
      heim

he·mo·ca·ther·e·sis

he·mo·cath·er·et·ic

He·moc·cult

Hem·oc·cult II

he·mo·chro·ma·to·sis

he·mo·chro·ma·tot·ic

he·mo·chrome

he·mo·chro·mo·gen
    hemoglobin h.

he·mo·cla·sis

he·mo·clas·tic

he·mo·con·cen·tra·tion

he·mo·co·nia

he·mo·co·ni·o·sis

he·mo·cry·os·co·py

he·mo·cul·ture

he·mo·cyte

he·mo·cy·to·blast

he·mo·cy·to·blas·to·ma

he·mo·cy·to·ca·ther·e·sis

he·mo·cy·to·ma

he·mo·cy·tom·e·ter

he·mo·cy·tom·e·try

he·mo·cy·to·pha·gia

he·mo·cy·to·phag·ic

he·mo·cy·to·poi·e·sis

he·mo·cy·to·trip·sis

he·mo·di·ag·no·sis

he·mo·di·al·y·sis

he·mo·di·lu·tion

he·mo·dy·nam·ic

he·mo·dy·nam·ics

he·mo·dys·tro·phy

he·mo·fus·cin

he·mo·gen·e·sis

he·mo·gen·ic

he·mo·glo·bin
    h. A
    h. A_{1c}
    h. A_2
    h. A_2 Adria
    h. A_2 Babinga
    h. A_2 Coburg
    h. A_2 Flatbush
    h. A_2 Indonesia
    h. A_2 Melbourne
    h. A_2 Roosevelt
    h. A_2 Sphakiá
    h. A_{Ia}
    h. A_{Ia2}
    h. A_{Ib}
    h. A_{Ic}
    h. A'_2
    h. Abraham Lincoln
    h. Abruzzo
    h. Agenogi
    h. Aida
    h. Alabama
    h. Alamo
    h. Alberta
    h. Altdorf

he·mo·glo·bin *(continued)*
- h. Anantharaj
- h. Andrew-Minneapolis
- h. Ankara
- h. Ann Arbor
- h. anti-Lepore
- h. Arlington Park
- h. Arya
- h. Atago
- h. Athens-Ga
- h. Atlanta
- h. Austin
- h. Avicenna
- h. B2
- h. Baltimore
- Bart's h.
- h. Baylor
- h. Beilinson
- h. Belfast
- h. Beograd
- h. Bethesda
- h. Beth Israel
- h. Bibba
- h. Bicêtre
- h. Böras
- h. Boyle Heights
- h. Brigham
- h. Bristol
- h. British Columbia
- h. Bryn Mawr
- h. Bucuresti
- h. Buenos Aires
- h. Bugines-X
- h. Burke
- h. Bushwick
- h. C
- h. C Georgetown
- h. C Harlem
- h. C Ziguinchor
- h. CC
- h. Camden
- h. Camperdown
- h. carbamate
- h. Caribbean
- h. Casper
- h. Castilla
- h. Chad
- h. Chapel Hill

he·mo·glo·bin *(continued)*
- h. Chesapeake
- h. Chiapas
- h. Chiba
- h. Christchurch
- h. Cochin-Port Royal
- h. Constant Spring
- h. Coventry
- h. Cranston
- h. Crete
- h. Creteil
- h. D
- h. D Bushman
- h. D Chicago
- h. D Ibadan
- h. D Iran
- h. D North Carolina
- h. D Ouled Rabah
- h. D Portugal
- h. D Punjab
- h. D St. Louis
- h. D Washington
- h. Dakar
- h. Danesgah-Tehran
- h. Deaconess
- h. Deer Lodge
- h. Denmark Hill
- deoxygenated h.
- h. Detroit
- h. Dhofar
- h. Djelfa
- h. Drenthe
- h. Duarte
- h. Dunn
- h. E
- h. E Saskatoon
- h. Edmonton
- h. Egypt
- h. Etobicoke
- h. F
- h. F Aleksandra
- h. F Auckland
- h. F Carlton
- h. F Dickinson
- h. F Hull
- h. F Jamaica
- h. F Kenya

he·mo·glo·bin *(continued)*
- h. F Kuala Lumpur
- h. F Malaysia
- h. F Malta-I
- h. F Melbourne
- h. F Poole
- h. F Port Royal
- h. F Texas-I
- h. F Texas-II
- h. F Ube
- h. F Victoria Jubilee
- h. F_I
- h. Fannin-Lubbock
- "fast" h's
- fetal h.
- h. FM Osaka
- h. Fort de France
- h. Fort Gordon
- h. Fort Worth
- h. Freiburg
- h. G
- h. G Accra
- h. G Audhali
- h. G Azakuoli
- h. G Bristol
- h. G Chinese
- h. G Copenhagen
- h. G Coushatta
- h. G Ferrara
- h. G Galveston
- h. G Georgia
- h. G Hong Kong
- h. G Honolulu
- h. G Hsi-Tsou
- h. G Knoxville-1
- h. G Makassar
- h. G Norfolk
- h. G Pest
- h. G Philadelphia
- h. G Port Arthur
- h. G San Jose
- h. G Saskatoon
- h. G Singapore
- h. G Szuhu
- h. G Taegu
- h. G Taichung
- h. G Taipei
- h. G Taiwan Ami

he·mo·glo·bin *(continued)*
- h. G Texas
- h. G Waimanalo
- h. Garden State
- h. Gavello
- h. Genova
- h. Gifu
- glycosylated h.
- h. Gothenburg
- Gower h.
- h. Gower 2
- h. Grady
- h. Gun Hill
- h. H
- h. Hacettepe
- h. Hamadan
- h. Hammersmith
- h. Handsworth
- h. Hasharon
- h. Heathrow
- h. Helsinki
- h. Henri Mondor
- h. Hijiyama
- h. Hikari
- h. Hikoshima
- h. Hirosaki
- h. Hirose
- h. Hiroshima
- h. Hofu
- homozygous h. (C, D, or E)
- h. Hope
- h. Hopkins-I
- h. Hopkins-II
- h. Hörlein-Weber
- h. Hoshida
- h. Hsin Chu
- h. I
- h. I Burlington
- h. I High Wycombe
- h. I Interlaken
- h. I Philadelphia
- h. I Skamania
- h. I Texas
- h. I Toulouse
- h. Icaria
- h. Indianapolis
- h. Inkster
- h. Istanbul

he·mo·glo·bin *(continued)*
   h. J
   h. J Abidjan
   h. J Aljezur
   h. J Altgeld Gardens
   h. J Baltimore
   h. J Bangkok
   h. J Bari
   h. J Birmingham
   h. J Broussais
   h. J Buda
   h. J Cairo
   h. J Calabria
   h. J Camagüay
   h. J Cambridge
   h. J Capetown
   h. J Chicago
   h. J Cosenza
   h. J Cubujuqui
   h. J Georgia
   h. J Guantanamo
   h. J Habana
   h. J Honolulu
   h. J Iran
   h. J Ireland
   h. J Kaohsiung
   h. J Korat
   h. J Kurosh
   h. J Lome
   h. J Manado
   h. J Medellin
   h. J Meerut
   h. J Meinung
   h. J Norfolk
   h. J Nyanza
   h. J Oxford
   h. J Paris-I
   h. J Paris-II
   h. J Rajappen
   h. J Rambam
   h. J Rovigo
   h. J Sardegna
   h. J Sicilia
   h. J Singapore
   h. J Taichung
   h. J Tongariki
   h. J Toronto
   h. J Trinidad

he·mo·glo·bin *(continued)*
   h. Jackson
   h. Jenkins
   h. K
   h. K Cameroon
   h. K Ibadan
   h. K Woolwich
   h. Kagoshima
   h. Kansas
   h. Karatsu
   h. Kempsey
   h. Kenwood
   h. Kenya
   h. Khartoum
   h. Knossos
   h. Kóos
   h. Köln
   h. Korle Bu
   h. Korura
   h. Koya Dora
   h. L
   h. L Ferrara
   h. L Gaslini
   h. L Persian Gulf
   h. Legnano
   h. Leiden
   h. Leipzig
   h. Lepore
   h. Lepore-Baltimore
   h. Lepore-Boston
   h. Lepore-Hollandia
   h. Lepore-Washington
   h. Leslie
   h. Little Rock
   h. Louisville
   h. Lufkin
   h. Lyon
   h. M
   h. M Akita
   h. M Arhus
   h. M Boston
   h. M Chicago
   h. M Emory
   h. M Erlangen
   h. M Hida
   h. M Hyde Park
   h. M Iwate
   h. M Kankakee

he·mo·glo·bin *(continued)*
   h. M Kiskunhalas
   h. M Kurume
   h. M Milwaukee-I
   h. M Oldenburg
   h. M Osaka
   h. M Radom
   h. M Saskatoon
   h. McKees Rocks
   h. Madrid
   h. Mahidol
   h. Malmö
   h. Manitoba
   h. Matsue-Oki
   mean corpuscular h.
   h. Memphis
   h. Mequon
   h. Mexico
   h. Michigan
   h. Miyada
   h. Mizuho
   h. Moabit
   h. Mobile
   h. Montgomery
   h. Moskva
   h. Mugino
   muscle h.
   h. N
   h. N Baltimore
   h. N Cosenza
   h. N Memphis
   h. N New Haven
   h. N Seattle
   h. Nagasaki
   h. Nancy
   h. New York
   h. Newcastle
   h. Nigeria
   h. Nishike
   h. Niteroi
   h. North Shore
   h. Nottingham
   h. Novi Sad
   h. O
   h. O Arab
   h. O Congo
   h. O Indonesia
   h. O Nilotic

he·mo·glo·bin *(continued)*
   h. O Padova
   h. Oak Ridge
   h. Ocho Rios
   h. Okaloosa
   h. Oliviere
   h. Olmsted
   h. Olympia
   h. Osler
   h. Osu Christiansborg
   h. Ottawa
   oxidized h.
   oxygenated h.
   h. P Congo
   h. P Galveston
   h. P Nilotic
   h. Parchman
   h. Persepolis
   h. Perth
   h. Petah Tikva
   h. Peterborough
   h. Philly
   h. Pontoise
   h. Portland
   h. Pôrto Alegre
   h. Port Philip
   h. Potomac
   h. Prato
   h. Presbyterian
   h. Providence
   h. Pyrgos
   pyridoxylated stroma-free
      h.
   h. Q
   h. Q India
   h. Q Iran
   h. Q Thailand
   h. Quong Sze
   h. Radcliffe
   h. Rahere
   h. Rainier
   h. Raleigh
   h. Rampa
   reduced h.
   h. Richmond
   h. Riverdale-Bronx
   h. Riyadh
   h. Rothchild

he·mo·glo·bin *(continued)*
- h. Rush
- h. Russ
- h. S
- h. S Travis
- h. Sabine
- h. St. Antoine
- h. St. Claude
- h. St. Etienne
- h. St. Louis
- h. St. Lukes
- h. Saki
- h. San Diego
- h. San Francisco
- h. Santa Ana
- h. Savannah
- h. Sawara
- h. Seal Rock
- h. Sealy
- h. Seattle
- h. Serbia
- h. Setif
- h. Shepherds Bush
- h. Sherwood Forest
- h. Shimonoseki
- h. Siam
- sickle h.
- h. Sinai
- h. Singapore
- h. Siriraj
- "slow" h's
- h. Sögn
- h. Southhampton
- h. Spanish Town
- h. Stanleyville-I
- h. Stanleyville-II
- h. Strasbourg
- stroma-free h.
- h. Strumica
- h. Suan Dok
- h. Sunshine Seth
- h. Suresnes
- h. Sydney
- h. Syracuse
- h. Ta-li
- h. Tacoma
- h. Tagawa-I
- h. Tagawa-II

he·mo·glo·bin *(continued)*
- h. Tak
- h. Tampa
- h. Tarrant
- h. Thailand
- h. Titusville
- h. Tochigi
- h. Tokuchi
- h. Torino
- h. Tours
- h. Tübingen
- h. Ty Gard
- h. Ube-1
- h. Ube-2
- h. Ube-4
- h. Umi
- unstable h.
- h. Uppsala
- h. Vaasa
- h. Vancouver
- h. Vanderbilt
- h. Vicksburg
- h. Volga
- h. Waco
- h. Wayne
- h. Wien
- h. Willamette
- h. Winnipeg
- h. Wood
- h. Yakima
- h. Yatsushiro
- h. York
- h. Yoshizuka
- h. Ypsilanti
- h. Yukuhashi-I
- h. Yukuhashi-II
- h. Zambia
- h. Zürich

he·mo·glo·bin·at·ed

he·mo·glo·bin·emia

he·mo·glo·bin·ol·y·sis

he·mo·glo·bin·om·e·ter

he·mo·glo·bin·om·e·try

he·mo·glo·bin·op·a·thy

he·mo·glo·bino·pep·sia

he·mo·glo·bi·nous

he·mo·glo·bin/spec·trin

he·mo·glo·bin·uria
    march h.
    paroxysmal cold h.
    paroxysmal nocturnal h.
    (PNH)

he·mo·gram

he·mo·his·tio·blast

he·mo·ki·ne·sis

he·mo·ki·net·ic

he·mol·o·gy

he·mo·lymph

he·mo·lymph·an·gi·o·ma

he·mol·y·sate

he·mol·y·sin
    alpha h.
    bacterial h.
    beta h.
    heterophile h.
    hot-cold h.
    immune h.

he·mol·y·sis
    contact h.
    immune h.
    impact h.
    mechanical h.
    passive h.

he·mo·lyt·ic

he·mo·lyz·a·ble

he·mo·ly·za·tion

he·mo·lyze

he·mom·e·ter

he·mom·e·try

he·mo·nec·tin

he·mo·path·ic

he·mo·pa·thol·o·gy

he·mop·a·thy

he·mo·pex·in

he·mo·phage

he·mo·phago·cyte

he·mo·phago·cy·to·sis

he·mo·phil·ia
    h. A
    h. B
    h. B Chapel Hill
    h. B Leyden
    h. B Oxford
    h. B Seattle
    h. B, Bm variant
    h. B, common variant
    B_M h.
    h. C
    classical h.
    vascular h.

he·mo·phil·i·ac

he·mo·phil·ic

he·mo·phil·i·oid

he·mo·phthi·sis

he·mo·plas·tic

he·mo·poi·e·sic

he·mo·poi·e·sis

he·mo·poi·et·ic

he·mo·poi·e·tin

he·mo·pre·cip·i·tin

he·mop·so·nin

He·mo·Quant

he·mo·rhe·ol·o·gy

he·mor·rhage
    colorectal h.
    fibrinolytic h.
    spontaneous h.

he·mor·rhe·ol·o·gy

he·mo·sta·sia

he·mo·sta·sis

he·mo·ther·a·peu·tics

he·mo·ther·a·py

he·mo·tox·ic

he·mo·trop·ic

Hep·a·lean

hep·a·ran sul·fate

hep·a·rin
low molecular weight h.

hep·a·rin·emia

Hep·a·rin Leo

hep·a·tec·to·my

hep·a·to·blas·to·ma

hep·a·to·car·cin·o·gen

hep·a·to·car·ci·no·gen·e·sis

hep·a·to·car·cin·o·gen·ic

hep·a·to·car·ci·no·ma

hep·a·to·cho·lan·gio·car·ci·
no·ma

hep·a·to·ma
malignant h.

hep·a·to·meg·a·ly

hep·a·top·a·thy
paraneoplastic h.

hep·a·to·por·phy·rin

hep·a·to·tox·ic

hep·a·to·tox·i·ci·ty

hep·a·to·tox·in

Hep3B (hepatoma) cell line

HepG2 (hepatoma) cell line

hep·to·glo·bin

hep·to·glo·bin·emia

Her·man·sky
H.-Pudlak syndrome

Hers
H. disease

het·ero·ge·ne·i·ty
regional h.

het·ero·phil

het·ero·phile

het·ero·phil·ic

Hex·a·CAF
hexamethylmelamine, cy-
clophosphamide, doxoru-
bicin, and 5-fluorouracil

hexa·meth·yl·mel·amine

hexa·meth·yl·meth·yl·amine

hexo·ki·nase

hexo·ki·nase de·fic·ien·cy

hex·os·amin·i·dase

HF
hyperfractionation

HFX
hyperfractionation

H (histocompatibility) gene

HGs
hematogones

5-HIAA
5-hydroxyindoleacetic acid

HI (hemagglutination
inhibition) as·say

hi·a·tus
h. leukemicus

hi·ber·no·ma

Hick·man
H. catheter
H. subcutaneous port

hi·drad·e·noides

hi·drad·e·no·ma

Hi·ga·shi
    Chédiak-H. anomaly
    Chédiak-H. disease
    Chédiak-H. syndrome
    Chédiak-Steinbrinck-H.
     anomaly

high-grade

HIL-3 cell

hi·ru·din

Hi·ru·do
    H. medicinalis

His·ma·nal

his·tam·i·ne·mia

His·tan·til

His·ter·one

his·tio·blast

his·tio·cyte
    wandering h's

his·tio·cyt·ic

his·tio·cy·to·ma
    fibrous h.
    malignant fibrous h.

his·tio·cy·to·ma·to·sis

his·tio·cy·to·sis
    adult h.
    regressing atypical h.
    h. X

his·ti·o·ma
    H's cells

his·to·com·pa·ti·bil·i·ty

his·to·com·pat·i·ble

his·to·cyte

his·to·gen·e·sis

his·to·in·com·pat·i·bil·i·ty

his·to·in·com·pat·i·ble

his·tol·o·gy
    bone marrow h.

his·to·ma

his·to·mor·pho·log·ic

His·to·paque
    H.-1077
    H.-1119

his·to·pa·thol·o·gy

HI (hemagglutination
    inhibition) test

HIV
    human immunodeficiency
    virus

H-2K^b gene

HLA-A lo·cus

HLA antigens

HLA-B lo·cus

HLA-C lo·cus

HLA-D lo·cus

HLA-DP lo·cus

HLA-DQ lo·cus

HLA-DR lo·cus

HLA fre·quen·cy

HLA-MB lo·cus

HLA-MT lo·cus

HLA-SB lo·cus

HLA-Te lo·cus

HLA typ·ing

HL-60 cell

HL-60 cell line

HMM
    hexamethylmelamine

Hmm
    hexamethymelamine

HMR
    histiocytic medullary re-
    ticulosis

HMWK
    high molecular weight ki-
      ninogen

HMW (high molecular weight)
ki·nin·o·gen

HN2
    nitrogen mustard
    mechlorethamine

HNPCC
    hereditary nonpolyposis
      colon cancer

HOAP-Bleo
    cytarabine, vincristine,
      doxorubicin, prednisone,
      and bleomycin

hoarse·ness

Hodg·kin
    H's disease
    H's ganglion
    H's lymphoma
    H's sarcoma
    non-H's lymphomas
    Reed-H. disease

hol·o·an·ti·gen

Ho·mer Wright
    Homer Wright rosette

hom·ing

hom·ing-as·so·ci·at·ed

ho·mo·body

ho·mo·cys·te·ine

ho·mo·graft

ho·mol·o·gous

ho·mol·o·gy

ho·mo·va·nil·lic acid

Hon·vol

HOP
    doxorubicin, vincristine,
      and prednisone

Hop·kins
    H.-Cole reaction

hor·mone
    adrenocorticotropic h.
    antidiuretic h.
    antitumor h.
    growth h. (GH)
    growth hormone releasing
      h. (GH-RH)
    luteinizing hormone re-
      leasing h. (LH-RH)
    thyroid h's
    thyroid-stimulating h.
      (TSH)

Hor·te·ga
    H. cell tumor

HOS (osteosarcoma) cell line

hos·pice

How·ell
    H's method
    H's test

HP
    hyperplastic polyp

H.P. Ac·thar Gel

HpD
    hepatoporphyrin

HPLC
    high-pressure liquid chro-
      matography
    high-performance liquid
      chromatography

HSC
    Hand-Schüller-Christian
      disease

H69 small cell lung carcinoma
cell line

H128 small cell lung
carcinoma cell line

Hsp
    heat shock protein

HSP70 gene

HSR
    hypersensitivity reaction

5-HT
    5-hydroxytryptamine (se-
    rotonin)

5HT
    5-hydroxytryptamine (se-
    rotonin)

HU
    hydroxyurea

Hu·ber
    H. needle

Hu·ët
    Pelger-H. nuclear anomaly
    pseudo–Pelger-H. anomaly

Hürth·le
    H. cell adenoma
    H. cell carcinoma
    H. cell neoplasia
    H. cell tumor

HUT 78 (T cell lymphoma) cell
line

Hutch·in·son
    melanotic freckle of H.

Hutch·i·son
    H. syndrome
    H. type

hy·a·lo·mere

Hy·bo·lin de·ca·no·ate

hy·brid·iza·tion
    nucleic acid h.
    Southern h.

hy·brid·o·ma

hy·da·tid·i·form

Hy·del·tra·sol

Hy·del·tra T.B.A.

Hy·drea

hy·dre·mia

hy·dro·car·bon
    carcinogenic h.
    polycyclic aromatic h.

hy·dro·chlo·ro·thi·a·zide
    amiloride and h.
    spironolactone and h.
    triamterene and h.

hy·dro·cor·ti·sone

Hy·dro·cor·tone ac·e·tate

Hy·dro·cor·tone phos·phate

hy·dro·cys·tad·e·no·ma

hy·dro·mor·phone

4-hy·dro·per·oxy·cy·clo·
phos·pha·mide (4-HC)

hy·dro·phago·cy·to·sis

hy·dro·thio·ne·mia

Hy·drox·a·cen

hy·droxy·chlo·ro·quine

hy·droxy·co·bal·a·min

hy·droxy·dau·no·my·cin

12-hy·droxy·ei·co·sa·tet·ra·
eno·ic acid

12-hy·droxy·hep·ta·dec·a·
tri·eno·ic acid

hy·droxy·in·dole·ace·tic acid

5-hy·droxy·in·dole·ace·tic
acid

hy·droxy·per·oxy·cy·clo·
phos·pha·mide

hy·droxy·pro·ges·ter·one

5-hy·droxy·tryp·ta·mine

hy·droxy·urea

hy·droxy·zine

Hy·lu·tin

hyp·al·bu·min·emia

hy·per·al·bu·min·emia

hy·per·al·o·ne·mia

hy·per·al·pha·lipo·pro·tein·
emia

hy·per·am·i·no·ac·i·de·mia

hy·per·am·mo·ne·mia

hy·per·am·mo·ni·emia

hy·per·am·y·las·emia

hy·per·azo·te·mia

hy·per·be·ta·lipo·pro·tein·
emia

hy·per·bi·car·bo·nat·emia

hy·per·bil·i·ru·bin·emia

hy·per·cal·ce·mia

hy·per·cal·ci·ne·mia

hy·per·cal·ci·to·nin·emia

hy·per·cel·lu·lar·i·ty

hy·per·chlor·emia

hy·per·chlor·emic

hy·per·cho·les·ter·emia

hy·per·cho·les·ter·emic

hy·per·cho·les·ter·in·emia

hy·per·cho·les·ter·ol·emia

hy·per·cho·les·ter·ol·emic

hy·per·chro·mat·ic

hy·per·chro·ma·tism

hy·per·chro·me·mia

hy·per·chy·lo·mi·cron·emia

hy·per·co·ag·u·la·bil·i·ty
paraneoplastic h.

hy·per·co·ag·u·la·ble

hy·per·cor·ti·sol·ism

hy·per·cu·pre·mia

hy·per·cy·a·not·ic

hy·per·cy·the·mia

hy·per·cy·to·sis

hy·per·dip·loid

hy·per·dip·loi·dy

hy·per·elec·tro·ly·te·mia

hy·per·eo·sin·o·phil·ia

hy·per·epi·neph·rin·emia

hy·per·eryth·ro·cy·the·mia

hy·per·es·trin·emia

hy·per·es·trin·ism

hy·per·es·tro·gen·emia

hy·per·fer·re·mia

hy·per·fer·re·mic

hy·per·fer·ri·ce·mia

hy·per·fi·bri·no·ge·ne·mia

hy·per·frac·tion·a·tion
accelerated h.

hy·per·func·tion·ing

hy·per·gam·ma·glob·u·lin·
emia
monoclonal h.

hy·per·gas·trin·emia

hy·per·gia

hy·per·glob·u·lin·emia

hy·per·glu·ca·gon·emia

hy·per·gly·ce·mia

hy·per·glyc·er·i·de·mia

hy·per·glyc·er·i·de·mic

hy·per·guan·i·din·emia

hy·per·he·mo·glo·bin·emia

hy·per·hep·a·rin·emia

hy·per·im·mu·no·glob·u·lin·
emia
h. E

hy·per·in·su·lin·emia

hy·per·io·de·mia

hy·per·ka·le·mia

hy·per·ke·ton·emia

hy·per·lact·ac·i·de·mia

hy·per·lec·i·thin·emia

hy·per·leu·ko·cy·to·sis

hy·per·li·pe·mia

hy·per·lip·id·emia

hy·per·li·poid·emia
    acquired h.

hy·per·li·the·mia

hy·per·na·tre·mia

hy·per·neo·cy·to·sis

hy·per·neph·roid

hy·per·ne·phro·ma

hy·per·ni·tre·mia

hy·per·or·tho·cy·to·sis

hy·per·os·mo·lar·i·ty

hy·per·ox·emia

hy·per·para·thy·roid·ism
    ectopic h.

hy·per·pep·sin·emia

hy·per·phos·pha·ta·se·mia

hy·per·phos·pha·te·mia

hy·per·phos·pho·re·mia

hy·per·pla·sia
    angiofollicular lymph node
        h.
    atypical h.
    benign immunoblastic h.
    congenital virilizing adre-
        nal h.
    diffuse h.
    giant lymph node h.
    granulocytic h.

hy·per·pla·sia *(continued)*
    lymphoid h.
    megakaryocytic h.
    megaloblastic h.
    mixed h.
    normoblastic h.

hy·per·plas·mia

hy·per·poly·pep·tid·emia

hy·per·pro·in·su·lin·emia

hy·per·pro·lac·tin·emia

hy·per·pro·tein·emia

hy·per·py·re·mia

hy·per·re·nin·emia

hy·per·sal·emia

hy·per·se·cre·tion
    gastric h.

hy·per·seg·men·ta·tion
    hereditary h. of neutro-
        phils

hy·per·sero·to·ne·mia

hy·per·skeo·cy·to·sis

hy·per·sple·nism

hy·per·ten·sion
    paraneoplastic h.

hy·per·ther·mia
    induced h.
    interstitial h.
    local h.
    regional h.
    systemic h.
    whole-body h.

hy·per·throm·bin·emia

hy·per·to·nia
    h. polycythaemica

hy·per·u·ric·ac·i·de·mia

hy·per·uri·ce·mia

hy·per·uri·ce·mic

hy·per·vas·cu·lar

hy·per·vis·cos·i·ty

hy·per·vo·le·mia

hy·per·vo·le·mic

hy·po·al·bu·min·emia

hy·po·al·do·ster·on·emia

hy·po·al·o·ne·mia

hy·po·am·i·no·ac·i·de·mia

hy·po·be·ta·lipo·pro·tein·emia

hy·po·cal·ce·mia

hy·po·cal·ce·mic

hy·po·cel·lu·lar·i·ty

hy·po·chlor·emia

hy·po·chlor·emic

hy·po·chlo·rid·emia

hy·po·chlo·rous acid

hy·po·cho·les·te·re·mia

hy·po·cho·les·te·re·mic

hy·po·cho·les·ter·in·emia

hy·po·cho·les·ter·ol·emia

hy·po·cho·les·ter·ol·emic

hy·po·chro·ma·sia

hy·po·chro·me·mia
 idiopathic h.

hy·po·chro·mia

hy·po·chro·mic

hy·po·chro·sis

hy·po·ci·tre·mia

hy·po·co·ag·u·la·bil·i·ty

hy·po·co·ag·u·la·ble

hy·po·com·ple·men·te·mia

hy·po·com·ple·men·te·mic

hy·po·cu·pre·mia

hy·po·cy·the·mia

hy·po·cy·to·sis

hy·po·dip·loid

hy·po·elec·tro·ly·te·mia

hy·po·eo·sin·o·phil·ia

hy·po·ep·i·neph·rin·emia

hy·po·er·gia

hy·po·es·trin·emia

hy·po·es·tro·gen·emia

hy·po·fer·re·mia

hy·po·fi·brin·o·gen·emia
 hereditary h.

hy·po·frac·tion·a·tion

hy·po·gam·ma·glob·u·lin·emia
 acquired h.
 common variable h.
 congenital h.
 physiologic h.
 transient h. of infancy
 X-linked h.
 X-linked infantile h.

hy·po·glu·ca·gon·emia

hy·po·gly·ce·mia
 paraneoplastic h.

hy·po·gly·ce·mic

hy·po·gran·u·lat·ed

hy·po·gran·u·lo·cy·to·sis

hy·po·in·su·lin·emia

hy·po·ka·le·mia

hy·po·li·pe·mia

hy·po·lipo·pro·tein·emia

hy·po·lym·phe·mia

hy·po·mag·ne·se·mia

hy·po·na·tre·mia
 hyperlipemic h.

hy·po·neo·cy·to·sis

hy·po·ni·tre·mia

hy·po-or·tho·cy·to·sis

hy·po·pha·ryn·ge·al

hy·po·phar·ynx

hy·po·phos·pha·ta·sia

hy·po·phos·pha·te·mia
    familial h.

hy·po·phys·ec·to·my

hy·po·pla·sia
    bone marrow h.
    constitutional erythroid h.
    erythrocytic h.
    lymphocytic h.

hy·po·pro·tein·emia

hy·po·pro·throm·bin·emia
    hereditary h.

hy·po·re·nin·emia

hy·po·sa·le·mia

hy·po·seg·ment·ed

hy·po·skeo·cy·to·sis

hy·po·ten·sion
    paraneoplastic h.

hy·po·ther·mia
    induced h.

hy·poth·e·sis
    cascade h.

hy·poth·e·sis *(continued)*
    Goldie-Coldman h.
    log cell kill h.
    Norton-Simon h.
    two-hit h. of carcinogene-
        sis

hy·po·thio·cy·an·ous acid

hy·po·throm·bin·emia

hy·po·thy·roid·ism

hy·po·ure·mia

hy·po·vas·cu·lar

hy·po·vo·le·mia

hy·po·vo·le·mic

hy·po·xan·thine

hy·pox·ia
    anemic h.

Hy·pro·gest

Hy·pro·val P.A.

hys·te·rec·to·my
    modified radical h.
    radical h.
    radical abdominal h.
    total abdominal h.

hys·tero·car·ci·no·ma

hys·tero·myo·ma

Hy·zine-50

IA
  intra-arterial

I-al·pha-an·ti·tryp·sin

IARC
  International Agency for
  Research on Cancer

ICA
  ileocolic anastomosis

ICAM-1
  intracellular adhesion
  molecule

ICRF
  ICRF-157
  ICRF-159

ic·tero·ane·mia

ic·ter·us
  chronic familial i.
  congenital familial i.
  congenital hemolytic i.

ida·ru·bi·cin

iden·ti·fi·ca·tion
  immunohistochemical i.

id·i·ol·y·sin

id·io·tope

id·io·type
  cross-reactive i.
  private lymphoma i.
  shared i.

id·io·typ·ic

IF
  involved field (irradiation)

IFEX

IFN-α
  interferon-α

IFN-α2a
  interferon-α2a

IFN-α2b
  interferon-α2b

IFN-β
  interferon-β

IFN-γ
  interferon-γ

ifos·fa·mide

Ig
  immunoglobulin

IgA
  immunoglobulin A

IgA1
  immunoglobulin A1

IgA2
  immunoglobulin A2

IgD
  immunoglobulin D

IgE
  immunoglobulin E

IgG
  immunoglobulin G

IgG1
  immunoglobulin G1

IgG2
  immunoglobulin G2

IgG3
  immunoglobulin G3

IgG4
  immunoglobulin G4

IgM
  immunoglobulin M

IgM1
  immunoglobulin M1

IgM2
   immunoglobulin M2

I/i an·ti·gen

IL
   interleukin

IL-1
   interleukin-1

IL-1α
   interleukin-1α

IL-1β
   interleukin-1β

IL-2
   interleukin-2

IL-2β
   interleukin-2β

IL-3
   interleukin-3

IL-4
   interleukin-4

IL-5
   interleukin-5

IL-6
   interleukin-6

IL-7
   interleukin-7

IL-8
   interleukin-8

IL-9
   interleukin-9

il·e·os·to·my

il·o·prost

imag·ing
   magnetic resonance i.
     (MRI)
   MoAb i.
   monoclonal antibody i.
   radiologic i.
   three-dimensional mag-
     netic resonance i.

Imers·lund
   I.-Graesbeck syndrome

5-im·i·no·dau·no·my·cin

Imm·ther

im·mune

im·mu·ni·ty
   cellular i.
   host i.

im·mu·ni·za·tion
   active i.
   passive i.

im·mu·nize

im·mu·no·ad·ju·vant

im·mu·no·as·say
   enzyme i.

im·mu·no·bi·ol·o·gy

im·mu·no·blast

im·mu·no·blas·tic

im·mu·no·che·mo·ther·a·py

im·mu·no·com·pe·tence

im·mu·no·com·pe·tent

im·mu·no·com·pro·mised

im·mu·no·con·glu·ti·nin

im·mu·no·cyte

im·mu·no·cy·to·ad·her·ence

im·mu·no·cy·to·chem·i·cal

im·mu·no·cy·to·chem·is·try

im·mu·no·cy·to·ma

im·mu·no·de·fi·cien·cy
   combined i.
   common variable i.
   common variable unclassi-
     fiable i.
   i. with hyper-IgM
   severe combined i.
   i. with thymoma

im·mu·no·di·ag·no·sis

im·mu·no·dif·fu·sion
    radial i. (RID)

im·mu·no·elec·tro·pho·re·sis
    counter i.
    countercurrent i.
    crossed i.
    rocket i.

im·mu·no·flu·o·res·cence

im·mu·no·gen

im·mu·no·ge·net·ic

im·mu·no·ge·net·ics

im·mu·no·gen·ic

im·mu·no·ge·nic·i·ty

im·mu·no·glob·u·lin
    intravenous i.
    monoclonal i.
    secretory i. A
    surface i.
    thyroid-binding inhibitory
      i's (TBII)
    thyroid-stimulating i's
      (TSI)
    TSH-binding inhibitory i's
      (TBII)

im·mu·no·glob·u·lin·op·a·thy

im·mu·no·hem·a·tol·o·gy

im·mu·no·his·to·chem·i·cal

im·mu·no·his·to·chem·is·try

im·mu·no·his·to·flu·o·res·cence

im·mu·no·his·to·log·ic

im·mu·no·his·tol·o·gy

im·mu·no·in·com·pe·tent

im·mu·no·log·ic

im·mu·no·log·i·cal

im·mu·nol·o·gy
    transplantation i.

im·mu·no·mod·u·la·tor

im·mu·no·pa·thol·o·gy

im·mu·nop·a·thy
    familial i.

im·mu·no·per·ox·i·dase

im·mu·no·phe·no·type

im·mu·no·phe·no·typ·ing

im·mu·no·pre·cip·i·ta·tion

im·mu·no·pro·lif·er·a·tive

im·mu·no·ra·dio·met·ric

im·mu·no·ra·di·om·e·try

im·mu·no·re·ac·tant

im·mu·no·re·ac·tion

im·mu·no·re·ac·tive

im·mu·no·re·ac·tiv·i·ty

im·mu·no·reg·u·la·tion

im·mu·no·re·spon·sive·ness

im·mu·no·se·lec·tion

im·mu·no·stain

im·mu·no·stain·ing

im·mu·no·stim·u·la·tion

im·mu·no·sup·pres·sant

im·mu·no·sup·pres·sion

im·mu·no·sup·pres·sive

im·mu·no·sur·veil·lance

im·mu·no·ther·a·py
    active i.
    active nonspecific i.
    active specific i.
    adjuvant i.
    adoptive i.
    local i.
    passive i.

im·mu·no·tox·in
    anti-TAP-72 i.

im·mu·no·tox·in *(continued)*
    CD5-T lymphocyte i.
    HD37-SAP i.
    HD39-SAP i.
    LFA-1 i.
    STI-RTA i. (SR 44163)

im·mu·no·trans·fu·sion

ImmuRAIT

im·pi·la·tion

im·plant
    tumor i.

IM·PLAN·TO·FIX port

im·pox
    immunoperoxidase

ImuVert

IMVP-16
    ifosfamide, methotrexate,
        etoposide, and leukovorin

INC
    inside-the-needle catheter

in·clu·sion
    leukocyte i's

in·co·ag·u·la·bil·i·ty

in·co·ag·u·la·ble

in·con·ti·nence
    bladder i.
    bowel i.

in·den·iza·tion

in·dex *pl.* in·dex·es, in·di·ces
    antitryptic i.
    Arneth i.
    Broders' i.
    erythrocyte i's
    Karnofsky i.
    Ki-67 i.
    opsonic i.
    phagocytic i.

In·di·a·na Uni·ver·si·ty reg·
    i·men (for testicular cancer)

In·di·a·na Uni·ver·si·ty
    stag·ing (for testicular
    cancer)

in·di·can·emia

in·di·um
    i. In 111 oxyquinoline

in·do·meth·a·cin

in·dox·yl·emia

in·duc·tion
    immunological i.
    magnetic loop i.
    remission i.
    i. therapy
    tolerance i.

in·farc·tion
    splenic i.

in·fec·tion
    opportunistic i.

in·fi·del·i·ty
    lineage i.

in·fil·trate
    cellular i.
    localized i.
    pulmonary i.

in·fil·trat·ing

in·fil·tra·tion
    i. of bone marrow
    diffuse i.
    multifocal i.
    tumor i.

in·flam·ma·tion

In·fu·med pump

In·fu·med 200 pump

in·fun·dib·u·lo·ma

In·fu·said Mi·cro·port

In·fus·aid pump

In·fu·sa·port

in·fu·sion
    hepatic artery i.
    intra-arterial i.
    multivitamin i.

In·fu·sor pump

in·hi·bi·tion
    allogenic i.

in·hib·i·tor
    alpha$_2$ plasma i.
    C$\overline{1}$ i. (C$\overline{1}$ INH)
    C1 esterase i.
    circulating i.
    extrinsic pathway i. (EPI)
    fibrinolytic i.
    I-protein C i.
    leukemia-associated i.
    lipoprotein-associated i.
    lipoprotein-associated co-
      agulation i. (LACI)
    membrane attack complex
      i. (MAC INH)
    mitosis i.
    mitotic i.
    plasma i.
    α_2 plasmin i.
    platelet i.
    plasminogen activator i.
      (PAI)
    polyamine i.
    prostaglandin i.
    serine protease i.
    stem cell i.
    thrombin i.
    tissue factor i.

ini·ti·a·tion

in·jec·tion
    epinephrine i.
    intracavernous i.
    phenylephrine i.

in·ju·ry
    ischemia-reperfusion i.

In(Lu) gene

in·nid·i·a·tion

in·op·er·a·ble

in·o·se·mia

INSS
    International Staging Sys-
      tem (for neuroblastoma)

in·stil·la·tion
    intraperitoneal i.

in·su·li·no·ma
    malignant i.

in·su·lo·ma

in·te·grin
    beta-1 i.
    beta-2 i.

in·ten·si·fi·ca·tion
    chemotherapy i.
    crossover i.

in·ten·si·ty
    dose i.

in·ter·cel·lu·lar

in·ter·change
    Hamburger i.

in·ter·fer·on
    i.-α (IFN-α)
    i.-α2a (IFN-α2a)
    i.-α2b (IFN-α2b)
    i. alfa-2a
    i. alfa-2b
    i. alfa-n1
    i. alfa-n3
    alpha i.
    i.-β (IFN-β)
    beta i.
    epithelial i.
    fibroblast i.
    fibroepithelial i.
    i.-γ (IFN-γ)
    gamma i.
    immune i.
    leukocyte i.
    lymphoblastoid alpha i.
    i. recombinant
    recombinant alpha i.

in·ter·fer·on *(continued)*
    recombinant beta i.
    type I i.
    type II i.

in·ter·leu·kin
    i.-1 (IL-1)
    i.-1α(IL-1α)
    i.-1β (IL-1β)
    i.-2 (IL-2)
    i.-2β (IL-2β)
    i.-3 (IL-3)
    i.-4 (IL-4)
    i.-5 (IL-5)
    i.-6 (IL-6)
    i.-7 (IL-7)
    i.-8 (IL-8)
    i.-9 (IL-9)
    i.-11 (IL-10)
    i.-12 (IL-11)
    i. recombinant

In·ter·na·tion·al Agen·cy for Re·search on Can·cer

In·ter·na·tion·al Nor·mal·ized Ra·tio

In·ter·na·tion·al Sen·si·tiv·i·ty In·dex

In·ter·na·tion·al Union Against Can·cer

in·ter·phase

in·ter·po·si·tion
    colon i.

in·ter·val
    disease-free i.
    progression-free i.

in·ter·ven·tion
    dietary i.

in·tra-ar·te·ri·al

in·tra·cav·i·tary

in·tra·cra·ni·al

in·tra·eryth·ro·cyt·ic

in·tra·he·pat·ic

in·tra·leu·ko·cyt·ic

in·tra·mu·co·sal

in·tra·oc·u·lar

In·tra·sil catheter

in·tra·ve·nous

in·tron

In·tron A

in·tu·ba·tion
    intraluminal i.

in·va·sion
    local i.
    lymphatic i.
    lymphatic vessel i.
    microscopic i.
    pseudocarcinomatous i.
    tumor i.

in·va·sive

in·va·sive·ness
    level of i.
    microscopic i.

in·ver·sion
    chromosome i.
    paracentric i.
    pericentric i.

in·volve·ment
    bilateral i.
    lymph node i.
    soft tissue i.

io·de·mia

io·dine

io·do·de·oxy·uri·dine

io·do·pep·tide
    two-dimensional i.

io·do·phil·ia

Io·do·tope
    vascular i.

ion·o·my·cin

ion·o·phore

IP
   intraperitoneal

ipro·pla·tin

I-pro·tein

IPT
   inflammatory pseudotumor

IRA
   ileorectal anastomosis

IRB
   immunoreactive bead

IRF-1
   interferon response factor 1

IRF-2
   interferon response factor 2

iri·tis
   leukemic i.

iron
   i. dextran
   i.-polysaccharide

ir·ra·di·a·tion
   abdominal i.
   boost i.
   charged-particle i.
   cranial i.
   electron-beam i.
   extended field i.
   external beam i.
   field i.
   hemibody i.
   hyperfractionated i.
   interstitial i.
   inverted-Y i.
   involved field i.
   local i.
   mantle field i.
   mantle-paraaortic-splenic
    i.
   neutron i.
   partial-brain i.
   prophylactic i.
   prophylactic cranial i.
   splenic i.
   subtotal lymphoid i.

ir·ra·di·a·tion *(continued)*
   therapeutic i.
   total body i.
   total lymphoid i.
   total nodal i.
   whole-brain i.

iso·ag·glu·ti·na·tion

iso·ag·glu·ti·nin

iso·an·ti·body

iso·an·ti·gen

iso·chro·mo·some

iso·cy·tol·y·sin

iso·dense

iso·en·zyme
   Regan i.

iso·ge·ne·ic

iso·graft

iso·hem·ag·glu·ti·na·tion

iso·hem·ag·glu·ti·nin

iso·he·mol·y·sin

iso·he·mol·y·sis

iso·he·mo·lyt·ic

iso·hy·dric

iso·in·tense

iso·la·tion
   reverse i.

iso·leu·ko·ag·glu·ti·nin

isol·o·gous

iso·plas·tic

iso·pro·pyl-benz·an·thra·cene

iso·pro·te·re·nol

iso·throm·bo·ag·glu·ti·nin

iso·trans·plant

iso·trans·plan·ta·tion

iso·tret·i·noin

iso·type

iso·typ·ic

ITP
    idiopathic thrombocyto-
        penic purpura

IUdR
    iododeoxyduridine

IV
    intravenous

IVGG
    intravenous immunoglobu-
        lin

Ivy
    I's method
    I. technique

Ja·cob
  J's ulcer

Jan·ský
  J's classification

Jap·a·nese fol·lic·u·lar lym·phoma

Jass
  J. staging (for rectal carcinoma)

jaun·dice
  acholuric familial j.
  chronic acholuric j.
  congenital acholuric j.
  familial acholuric j.
  hemolytic j.
  obstructive j.
  painless j.

J82 cell

J (joining) chain

Jeg·hers
  Peutz-J. polyp
  Peutz-J. syndrome

Jen·ner
  J's stain

JIM (myeloma cell) cell line

jog·ging

joint
  bleeders' j.
  hemophilic j.

Jones
  Price-J. curve
  Price-J. method

Jo·sephs
  J.-Diamond-Blackfan syndrome

JP
  juvenile polyposis

JPA
  juvenile pilocytic astrocytoma

juice
  cancer j.

jun gene

Jung·hans
  Wolff-J. test

Kab·o·lin

Kah·ler
  K's disease

ka·le·mia

Kal·i·um Du·rules

kal·li·kre·in
  plasma k.

Ka·o·chlor

Ka·on

Kaon-Cl

Ka·po·si
  K's sarcoma
  pseudo-K. sarcoma

Kar·nof·sky
  K. index
  K. 422 lymphoma cell line

karyo·type

karyo·typ·ic

karyo·typ·ing

Ka·su·mi
  K.-1 AML cell line

Ka·to
  K's test

Ka·wa·sa·ki
  K. disease

Kay Ciel

Kay·ex·a·late

Kay·lix·ir

Kaz·nel·son
  K's syndrome

KB cell

K562 cell

KDO
  keto-deoxyoctonic acid

K-Dur

Keas·by
  K. tumor

Kell
  K. blood group

Kel·ling
  K's test

Kel·ly
  Patterson-K. syndrome

Ken·ny
  K. syndrome

ke·rat·i·no·cyte

ker·a·to·sis *pl.* ker·a·to·ses
  actinic k.
  solar k.

Ker·no·han
  K. classification (for astro-
    cytomas)

K562 eryth·ro·leu·ke·mia
  cell

K562 eryth·ro·leu·ke·mia
  cell line

Kes·trin Aq·ue·ous

Kes·trone-5

ke·to·con·a·zole

ke·to-de·oxy·oc·ton·ic acid

ke·to·ne·mia

ke·to·ste·roid
  3-k.
  17-k's

ke·to-tet·ra·hy·dro·phen·an·
  threne

Ke·to·trol

Key-Pred

KG-1 cell

K-G Elix·ir

KGN
    kininogen

Kidd
    K. blood group

K-Ide

Kid·ro·lase

Ki-67 in·dex

ki·nase
    GAP k.

ki·net·ics
    C2 k.
    cell k.
    gompertzian cell k.

ki·nin·o·gen
    high molecular weight k.
    HMW (high molecular
        weight) k.

KL-60 cell

Klei·hau·er
    K.-Betke test

K562 leu·ke·mia cell

K-Long

K-Lor

Klor-Con

Klor-Con/EF

Klor·vess

Klo·trix

K-Lyte

K-Lyte/Cl

KMOE eryth·ro·leu·ke·mia
    cell line

knife
    gamma k.

K-Norm

Ko·bert
    K's test

Kon·a·ki·on

Kost·mann
    K. neutropenia
    K's syndrome

K-Phen-50

K-Phos M. F.

K-Phos Neu·tral

K-Phos No. 2

K-*ras* on·co·gene

kre·bi·o·zen

krin·gle

Krom·pech·er
    K's carcinoma
    K's tumor

Kru·ken·berg
    K's tumor

KS
    Kaposi sarcoma

K-Tab

KU 812 cell line

Kul·chit·sky
    K.-cell carcinoma

Kupf·fer
    K. cell sarcoma

kVP
    kilovolts peak

LACI
　　lipoprotein-associated co-
　　　agulation inhibitor

lac·tate

lac·tate de·hy·dro·gen·ase

lac·tic de·hy·dro·gen·ase

lac·ti·ce·mia

lac·to·fer·rin

lac·to·gen
　　human placental l.
　　placental l.

Lac·tu·lax

lac·tu·lose

La·e·trile

LAF
　　laminar air flow (room)

LAG
　　lymphangiogram

L.A.E. 20

LAK
　　lymphokine-activated
　　　killer (cell)

lake

La·ki
　　L.-Lorand factor

LAM-1
　　leukocyte adhesion mole-
　　　cule-1

lam·i·nin

La·my
　　Maroteaux-L. syndrome

Lands·berg
　　Wintrobe and L.'s method

Land·stein·er
　　Donath-L. antibody

Lan·ger
　　L.-Giedion syndrome

lap·a·ros·co·py

lap·a·rot·o·my
　　second-look l.
　　staging l.

lar·yn·gec·to·my
　　horizontal supraglottic l.
　　supraglottic l.
　　total l.
　　vertical l.

la·ser
　　Nd:YAG l.
　　neodymium:YAG l.

Lau·rell
　　L. technique

law
　　Collin's l.
　　Virchow's l.

LB 84-1 cell line

LCA
　　leukocyte common antigen

L-CFC
　　leukemia colony-forming
　　　cell

L (light) chain

LCL
　　large cell lymphoma

LCSG
　　Lung Cancer Study Group

LD
　　lymphocyte-depleted
　　　Hodgkin's disease

Leach
　　L. phenotype

LECAM-1
leukocyte-endothelial cell
adhesion molecule-1

lec·i·thin·emia

lec·tin

leech
medicinal l.
Mexican l.

leio·myo·blas·to·ma

leio·myo·fi·bro·ma

leio·myo·ma
bizarre l.
epithelioid l.
vascular l.

leio·myo·sar·co·ma

Len·nert
L's lymphoma

len·tig·i·nes

len·tig·i·nous

len·ti·go *pl.* len·ti·gi·nes
l. maligna

Leon·ard
L. catheter

Le·pore
hemoglobin L.

lep·to·cyte

lep·to·cy·to·sis

Le·ser
L.-Trélat sign

le·sion
coin l.
immunoproliferative l.
isodense l.
neoplastic l.
paraneoplastic l.
pedunculated l.
polypoid l.
precancerous l.
premalignant l.

le·sion *(continued)*
sessile l.

LET
linear energy transfer

Let·ter·er
L.-Siwe disease

leu·co·cyte

leu·co·cy·to·sis

leu·co·vo·rin

leu·ka·phe·re·sis

leu·ke·mia
acute l.
acute lymphoblastic l.
(ALL)
acute lymphocytic l.
acute megakaryoblastic l.
acute monoblastic l.
(AMOL)
acute monocytic l.
acute myeloblastic l.
(AML)
acute myelocytic l.
acute myelogenous l.
acute myelomonocytic l.
acute nonlymphocytic l.
(ANLL)
acute prolymphocytic l.
acute promyelocytic l.
acute undifferentiated l.
adult T-cell l.
adult T-cell l./lymphoma
aleukemic l.
aleukocythemic l.
basophilic l.
B cell l.
bilineage l.
bilineal l.
biphenotypic l.
blast cell l.
central nervous system l.
chronic l.
chronic granulocytic l.
chronic lymphocytic l.
(CLL)

leu·ke·mia *(continued)*
    chronic myelocytic l.
    chronic myelocytic l. in
      metamorphosis
    chronic myelomonocytic l.
    chronic prolymphocytic l.
    cIg-positive acute lympho-
      cytic l.
    CNS l.
    congenital l.
    cranial nerve l.
    cutaneous l.
    embryonal l.
    eosinophilic l.
    extramedullary l.
    gastric l.
    genitourinary l.
    granulocytic l.
    hairy-cell l.
    hand mirror cell l.
    hemoblastic l.
    hemocytoblastic l.
    hepatic l.
    histiocytic l.
    hybrid l.
    leukopenic l.
    lymphatic l.
    lymphoblastic l.
    lymphocytic l.
    lymphogenous l.
    lymphoid l.
    lymphosarcoma cell l.
    M3 l.
    mast cell l.
    mediastinal l.
    megakaryoblastic l.
    megakaryocytic l.
    meningeal l.
    micromyeloblastic l.
    mixed-lineage l.
    monocytic l.
    myeloblastic l.
    myelocytic l.
    myelogenous l.
    myeloid l.
    myeloid granulocytic l.
    myelomonocytic l.
    Naegeli l.

leu·ke·mia *(continued)*
    neonatal l.
    null cell acute lympho-
      blastic l.
    pancreatic l.
    plasma cell l.
    plasmacytic l.
    prolymphocytic l.
    promyelocytic l.
    prostatic l.
    pulmonary l.
    refractory l.
    retinal l.
    Rieder cell l.
    Schilling's l.
    secondary l.
    stem cell l.
    subleukemic l.
    T-cell l.
    T-cell l./lymphoma
    T-cell acute lymphoblastic
      l.
    T-cell chronic lymphocytic
      l.
    testicular l.
    thyroid l.
    undifferentiated cell l.
    urinary tract l.

leu·ke·mic

leu·ke·mid

leu·ke·mo·gen

leu·ke·mo·gen·e·sis
    clonal l.

leu·ke·mo·gen·ic

leu·ke·moid

Leu·ker·an

Leu·kine

leu·ko·ag·glu·ti·nin

leu·ko·blas·to·sis

leu·ko·crit

leu·ko·cy·tal

leu·ko·cyte
    agranular l's
    basophilic l.
    endothelial l.
    eosinophilic l.
    granular l's (granulocytes)
    heterophilic l's
    hyaline l.
    lymphoid l's
    mast l.
    motile l.
    neutrophilic l.
    nongranular l's
    nonmotile l.
    polymorphonuclear l.
    polynuclear neutrophilic l.

leu·ko·cyte per·ox·i·dase

leu·ko·cy·the·mia

leu·ko·cyt·ic

leu·ko·cy·to·blast

leu·ko·cy·to·gen·e·sis

leu·ko·cy·toid

leu·ko·cy·tol·o·gy

leu·ko·cy·tol·y·sin

leu·ko·cy·tol·y·sis

leu·ko·cy·to·lyt·ic

leu·ko·cy·to·pe·nia

leu·ko·cy·toph·a·gy

leu·ko·cy·to·pla·nia

leu·ko·cy·to·poi·e·sis

leu·ko·cy·to·sis
    absolute l.
    agonal l.
    basophilic l.
    central nervous system l.
    mononuclear l.
    neutrophilic l.
    pathologic l.
    physiologic l.
    pure l.

leu·ko·cy·to·sis *(continued)*
    relative l.
    terminal l.
    toxic l.

leu·ko·cy·to·ther·a·py

leu·ko·cy·to·tox·ic·i·ty

leu·ko·cy·to·trop·ic

leu·ko·en·ceph·a·lop·a·thy

leu·ko·eryth·ro·blas·tic

leu·ko·eryth·ro·blas·to·sis

leu·ko·gram

leu·ko·ki·ne·sis

leu·ko·ki·net·ic

leu·ko·ki·net·ics

leu·ko·ki·nin

leu·ko·lym·pho·sar·co·ma

leu·kol·y·sin

leu·kol·y·sis

leu·ko·lyt·ic

leu·ko·mono·cyte

leu·ko·my·o·ma

leu·kon

leu·ko·pe·de·sis

leu·ko·pe·nia
    basophil l.
    basophilic l.
    congenital l.
    malignant l.
    neutrophilic l.
    pernicious l.

leu·ko·pe·nic

leu·ko·phago·cy·to·sis

leu·ko·pla·kia

leu·ko·poi·e·sis

leu·ko·poi·et·ic

leu·ko·poi·e·tin

leu·ko·pre·cip·i·tin

leu·ko·sar·co·ma

leu·ko·sar·co·ma·to·sis

leu·ko·sis *pl.* leu·ko·ses
  lymphoid l.
  myeloblastic l.
  myelocytic l.

leu·ko·sta·sis
  intracerebral l.

leu·ko·throm·bin

leu·ko·tox·ic

leu·ko·tox·ic·i·ty

leu·ko·tox·in

leu·ko·tri·ene

leu·pro·lide

lev·am·i·sole
  l. hydrochloride

lev·el
  carcinoembryonic antigen
    l.
  l. of invasiveness

Le·void

lev·or·pha·nol tar·trate

Le·vo·throid

le·vo·thy·rox·ine

Le·vox·ine

lev·u·los·emia

Le·vy
  L., Rowntree, and Mar-
    riott's method

Lew·is
  L. blood group
  L. phenomenon

Ley·den
  hemophilia B, L.

Ley·dig
  Sertoli-L. cell tumor

LFA-1 ad·he·sion mol·e·cule

LFA-3 ad·he·sion mol·e·cule

L929 (fibrosarcoma) cell line

LG
  lymphography

LGL
  large granular lymphocyte

LGL (large granular
  lymphocyte) syndrome

Lher·mitte
  L's sign

LHR
  lymphocyte homing recep-
    tor

LHRH
  luteinizing hor-
    mone–releasing hormone

Li
  L.-Fraumeni syndrome

li·chen
  l. myxedematosus

LIF
  leukemia inhibitory factor

Life·Port

li·gand
  c-*kit* l.
  cold l.

limb-spar·ing

Lim·u·lus
  L. amebocyte assay

Lin·berg
  Tikhor-L. operation

Lin·dau
  von Hippel-L. syndrome

Lind·qvist
  Fahraeus-L. effect

line
   AML-193 leukemic cell l.
   AML-WC (myelomonocy-
      tic) cell l.
   BCZ-91 (stem cell) l.
   BL3 (SCA-1$^+$ stem cell) l.
   BS-1 (stromal) cell l.
   BXL-40 (stromal) cell l.
   CESS cell l.
   C6 (glioma) cell l.
   CHP134 (neuroblastoma)
      cell l.
   Dami human megakaryo-
      cytic cell l.
   Daudi cell l.
   DS19-Sc9 (erythroleuke-
      mia) cell l.
   D2XRII (hematopoietic)
      cell l.
   EM2 (myeloid) cell l.
   EM3 (myeloid) cell l.
   FDC-P1 (myeloid) cell l.
   Hep3B (hepatoma) cell l.
   HepG2 (hepatoma) cell l.
   HL-60 cell l.
   HOS (osteosarcoma) cell l.
   H69 small cell lung carci-
      noma cell l.
   H128 small cell lung car-
      cinoma cell l.
   HUT 78 (T cell lymphoma)
      cell l.
   JIM (myeloma cell) cell l.
   K562 erythroleukemia cell
      l.
   Karpas 422 lymphoma cell
      l.
   Kasumi-1 AML cell l.
   KMOE erythroleukemia
      cell l.
   KU 812 cell l.
   LB 84-1 cell l.
   L929 (fibrosarcoma) cell l.
   L8057 (murine mega-
      karyoblast) cell l.
   LP-1 cell l.
   Lu-CSF-1 (lung tumor)
      cell l.

line *(continued)*
   MB-02 (erythroleukemia)
      cell l.
   MB-03 (megakaryoblastic)
      cell l.
   MG-63 (osteosarcoma) cell
      l.
   M20 (myelomonocytic) cell
      l.
   MO7E (myeloblast) cell l.
   MO7 (myeloid leukemia)
      cell l.
   NB4 cell l.
   NIH 3T3 (fibroblast) cell l.
   NKM-1 (myeloid) cell l.
   NOMO-1 cell l.
   OC-2008 (ovarian carci-
      noma) cell l.
   Ohngren's l.
   PBEI (Pre-B lymphoblast)
      cell l.
   PICC l.
   RC-1 (renal carcinoma)
      cell l.
   SId4656 (stromal) cell l.
   SK-MEL-37 (melanoma)
      cell l.
   SUP-M2 (large cell lym-
      phoma) cell l.
   suture l.
   Sydney l.
   TC-1 (stromal) cell l.
   THP-1 (monocytic leuke-
      mia) cell l.
   VT7 (megakaryocytic) cell
      l.

lin·e·age
   l. infidelity
   l. promiscuity

lin·o·le·ic acid

Lin-Trol

li·o·thy·ro·nine

li·o·trix

li·pe·mia

lip·id
   l. A
   l. X

lip·i·de·mia

lip·id·ic

Lip·io·dol

lipo·blas·to·ma

lipo·blas·to·ma·to·sis

lipo·chon·dro·ma

lipo·chro·me·mia

lipo·fi·bro·ma

lipo·he·mia

lip·oi·de·mia

li·po·ma
   l. arborescens
   l. capsulare
   l. cavernosum
   fat cell l., fetal
   l. fibrosum
   l. myxomatodes
   l. ossificans
   l. sarcomatodes
   telangiectatic l.
   l. telangiectodes

li·po·ma·toid

li·po·ma·tous

lipo·myo·he·man·gi·o·ma

lipo·my·o·ma

lipo·myx·o·ma

lipo·poly·sac·cha·ride

lipo·pro·tein-as·so·ci·at·ed

lipo·pro·tein·emia

lipo·sar·co·ma

lipo·some

li·pox·in

li·poxy·ge·nase
   platelet l.

li·quor *pl.* li·quors, li·quo·res
   l. sanguinis

li·the·mia

li·the·mic

lith·i·um
   l. carbonate

LL
   lymphoblastic leukemia

LMM
   lentigo maligna melanoma

LMP
   latent membrane protein

L8057 (murine
   megakaryoblast) cell line

LNH-80

LNH-84

lobe
   nuclear l.

lo·bec·to·my
   sleeve l.

Lo·cal·io
   L. operation

lo·cus *pl.* lo·ci, lo·ca
   FAP l.
   HLA-A l.
   HLA-B l.
   HLA-C l.
   HLA-D l.
   HLA-DP l.
   HLA-DQ l.
   HLA-DR l.
   HLA-MB l.
   HLA-MT l.
   HLA-SB l.
   HLA-Te l.

lo·mus·tine

Lo·pid

LOPP
  chlorambucil, vincristine, procarbazine, prednisone

Lo·rand
  Laki-L. factor

lor·at·a·dine

Lo·rel·co

Lo·sec

Lo·so·tron Plus

loss
  platelet l.

Los·sen
  L's rule

Lou·is-Bar
  L.-B. syndrome

lov·a·sta·tin

Lö·wen·stein
  Buschke-L. tumor

low-grade

Low·si·um

lox·o·ri·bine

LP
  lymphocyte-predominant Hodgkin's disease

L-PAM
  melphalan (L-phenylala-nine mustard)

LP-1 cell line

LPS
  lipopolysaccharide

LRD
  local regional disease

LS
  lymphosarcoma

LSA
  lymphosarcoma

LSA₂-L₂ (combined therapy regimen)

LSD
  Letterer-Siwe disease

L-S (Letterer-Siwe) disease

LTMC
  long-term marrow culture

Lu-CSF-1 (lung tumor) cell line

Lu·er-Lok cap

Lu·er-Lok nee·dle tip

lu·mi·ag·gre·gom·e·try

lum·pec·to·my

Lung Can·cer Study Group

Lu·pron

lu·pus
  l. anticoagulant
  l. erythematosus (LE)

lu·te·in
  serum l.

Lu·ther·an
  L. blood group

LV
  leucovorin
  leukovorin

Lv
  leucovorin
  leukovorin

LVB
  lomustine, vindesine, and bleomycin sulfate

LYDMA
  lymphocyte-determined membrane antigen

lym·phad·e·nec·to·my
  bilateral l.
  para-aortic l.
  regional l.

lym·phad·e·no·ma

lym·phad·e·nop·a·thy
    angioimmunoblastic l.
    angioimmunoblastic l.
      with dysproteinemia
      (AILD)
    immunoblastic l.
    superficial l.

lym·phad·e·no·sis

lym·phan·gi·og·ra·phy

lym·phan·gio·sar·co·ma

lym·phan·git·ic

lym·phan·gi·tis
    l. carcinomatosa

lym·pha·phe·re·sis

lym·phat·ic

lym·phe·de·ma
    postmastectomy l.

lymph·epi·the·li·o·ma

lym·pho·blast

lym·pho·blas·tic

lym·pho·blas·to·ma

lym·pho·blas·to·sis

lym·pho·cy·ta·phe·re·sis

lym·pho·cyte
    amplifier T-l.
    B l's
    bone marrow–derived l.
    cytotoxic T l's (CTL)
    l.-depleted
    killer l.
    large granular l's
    natural killer (NK) l.
    peripheral blood l.
    plasmacytoid l.
    l.-predominant
    Rieder's l.
    T l's
    thymus-dependent l's
    thymus-independent l's
    tumor-infiltrating l.

lym·pho·cyte *(continued)*
    tumor-infiltrating T l.

lym·pho·cyt·ic

lym·pho·cy·to·blast

lym·pho·cy·to·ma
    l. cutis

lym·pho·cy·to·pe·nia

lym·pho·cy·to·phe·re·sis

lym·pho·cy·to·poi·e·sis

lym·pho·cy·to·poi·et·ic

lym·pho·cy·tor·rhex·is

lym·pho·cy·to·sis
    monoclonal B cell l.
    reactive l.

lym·pho·cy·tot·ic

lym·pho·cy·to·tox·ic·i·ty

lym·pho·cy·to·tox·in

lym·pho·epi·the·li·al

lym·pho·epi·the·li·o·ma
    nasopharyngeal l.

lym·pho·gran·u·lo·ma
    l. malignum

lym·pho·gran·u·lo·ma·to·sis
    l. cutis
    l. maligna

lym·phog·ra·phy

lym·pho·his·tio·cyt·ic

lym·pho·his·tio·cy·to·sis
    erythrophagocytic l.
    familial l.

lym·pho·his·tio·plas·ma·cyt·ic

lym·phoid

lym·phoi·do·cyte

lym·pho·ken·tric

lym·pho·kine
    T cell–mediated l.
    tumor-infiltrating l's

lym·pho·kine-ac·ti·vat·ed

lym·pho·kine-spe·cif·ic

lym·pho·leu·ke·mia
    acute T-cell l.

lym·phol·y·sis
    cell-mediated l. (CML)

lym·pho·lyt·ic

lym·pho·ma
    adult T-cell l.
    adult T-cell leukemia/l.
    African l.
    African Burkitt's l.
    American Burkitt's l.
    anaplastic large-cell l.
    anorectal l.
    B cell l.
    B-cell monocytoid l.
    l. of bone
    Burkitt's l.
    cardiac l.
    centrocytic l.
    CNS l.
    colorectal l.
    composite l.
    l. of conjunctiva
    cutaneous l.
    cutaneous T-cell l.
    l. cutis
    diffuse l.
    diffuse aggressive l.
    diffuse immunoblastic l.
    diffuse intermediate lym-
        phocytic l.
    diffuse large-cell l.
    diffuse mixed small- and
        large-cell l.
    diffuse small cleaved-cell l.
    diffuse small noncleaved-
        cell l.
    endemic Burkitt's l.
    esophageal l.

lym·pho·ma (continued)
    extranodal non-Hodgkin's
        l.
    follicular l.
    follicular center cell l.
    follicular lymphocytic l.
    giant follicle l.
    giant follicular l.
    l. of heart
    histiocytic l.
    Hodgkin's l.
    immunoblastic l.
    intermediate lymphocytic
        l.
    Japanese follicular l.
    Ki-1 l.
    Ki-1 (CD30) large cell l.
    large cell l. (LCL)
    Lennert's l.
    lymphoblastic l.
    lymphocytic l.
    lymphocytic l., plasmacy-
        toid
    lymphocytic l., poorly dif-
        ferentiated
    lymphocytic l., well-differ-
        entiated
    malignant l.
    Mediterranean l.
    meningeal l.
    mixed lymphocytic-histio-
        cytic l.
    nasopharyngeal l.
    nodular l.
    nodular mixed l.
    noncleaved cell l.
    nonendemic Burkitt's l.
    non-Hodgkin's l's
    orbital l.
    peripheral T-cell l.
    pleomorphic l.
    pleomorphic peripheral T-
        cell l.
    primary l.
    renal l.
    Sézary l.
    sinonasal l.
    small B-cell l.

lym·pho·ma *(continued)*
    splenic l. with villous lym-
      phocytes
    T-cell l's.
    T-cell l., convoluted
    T-cell l., cutaneous
    T-cell leukemia/l.
    T-cell l., small lymphocytic
    U-cell (undefined) l.
    undifferentiated l.

lym·pho·ma·toid

lym·pho·ma·to·sis

lym·pho·ma·tous

lym·pho·myx·o·ma

lym·pho·pe·nia

lym·pho·plas·ma·phe·re·sis

lym·pho·poi·e·sis

lym·pho·poi·et·ic

lym·pho·pro·lif·er·a·tive

lym·pho·sar·co·ma
    fascicular l.
    sclerosing l.

lym·pho·sar·co·ma·to·sis

lym·pho·tax·is

lym·pho·tox·in

lym·phot·ro·phy

Lymph-Scan

Lynch
    L. syndrome (I and II)

LyP
    lymphomatoid papulosis

ly·sin
    beta l.

ly·sine

ly·sin·o·gen

ly·sis
    euglobulin clot l.
    hypotonic l.

Ly·so·dren

ly·so·gen

ly·so·gen·e·sis

ly·so·gen·ic

ly·so·ge·nic·i·ty

ly·so·ki·nase

ly·so·zyme

Lys-plas·min·o·gen

lyt·ic

M
mechlorethamine hydro-
chloride

MAb
monoclonal antibody

MABOP
mechlorethamine, doxoru-
bicin, bleomycin sulfate,
vincristine, and predni-
sone

MAC
methotrexate, dactinomy-
cin, and cyclophospha-
mide

MACC
methotrexate, doxorubicin,
cyclophosphamide, lo-
mustine

MAC INH
membrane attack complex
inhibitor

Mc·Ku·sick
diaphyseal chondrodyspla-
sia, M. type
metaphyseal chondrodys-
plasia, M. type

Mc·Neer
M. classification

MACOP-B
methotrexate, doxorubicin,
cyclophosphamide, vin-
cristine, prednisone, and
bleomycin sulfate

mac·ro·ad·e·no·ma

mac·ro·am·y·lase

mac·ro·am·yl·a·se·mia

mac·ro·am·yl·a·se·mic

mac·ro·cyte

mac·ro·cy·the·mia

mac·ro·cyt·ic

mac·ro·cy·to·sis

mac·ro·e·ryth·ro·blast

mac·ro·glob·u·lin
α_2-m.

mac·ro·glob·u·lin·emia
Waldenström's m.

mac·ro·leu·ko·blast

mac·ro·lym·pho·cyte

mac·ro·lym·pho·cy·to·sis

mac·ro·mono·cyte

mac·ro·my·elo·blast

mac·ro·nor·mo·blast

mac·ro·phage
armed m's
fixed m.
free m.
inflammatory m.

mac·ro·phago·cyte

ma·croph·a·gus

mac·ro·poly·cyte

mac·ro·pro·lac·ti·no·ma

mac·ro·pro·my·elo·cyte

Mac·ro·tec

mac·ro·throm·bo·cy·to·pe·
nia

MAF
macrophage activating
factor

Maf·fuc·ci
M. syndrome

ma·fos·fa·mide

mag·al·drate
m. and simethicone

mag·nes·emia

mag·ne·sia
    alumina and m.
    alumina, m., and calcium
        carbonate
    alumina, m., and simethi-
        cone
    calcium carbonate and m.
    calcium carbonate, m., and
        simethicone
    magnesium trisilicate, al-
        umina, and m.
    simethicone, alumina, cal-
        cium carbonate, and m.
    simethicone, alumina,
        magnesium carbonate,
        and m.

mag·ne·si·um
    alumina and m. carbonate
    alumina and m. trisilicate
    alumina, m. trisilicate,
        and sodium bicarbonate
    calcium and m. carbonates
    m. carbonate and sodium
        bicarbonate
    m. hydroxide
    m. oxide
    simethicone, alumina, m.
        carbonate, and magnesia
    m. sulfate
    m. trisilicate, alumina,
        and magnesia

Mag·ne·vist

main·te·nance

mal·ab·sorp·tion
    paraneoplastic m.

ma·lig·na

ma·lig·nan·cy
    borderline m.
    high-grade m.
    histiocytic m.
    low-grade m.
    lymphoid m.
    musculoskeletal m.
    occult primary m.

ma·lig·nan·cy *(continued)*
    postirradiation m.
    primary m.
    second m.
    T-cell m.
    underlying m.

ma·lig·nant

ma·lig·nin

Mal·in
    M. syndrome

Mal·mö
    M. polymorphism
    M. regimen

Mal·o·gen

Mal·o·gex

mam·mo·gram

mam·mog·ra·phy
    consultative m.
    diagnostic m.
    film-screen m.
    problem-solving m.
    screening m.

man·age·ment
    pain m.

man·dib·u·lec·to·my

man·gan·ese su·per·ox·ide
dis·mu·tase

ma·nip·u·la·tion
    adjuvant endocrine m.

Mar·chand
    M's cell

Mar·chi·a·fa·va
    M.-Micheli disease
    M.-Micheli syndrome

mar·gin
    anal m.
    distal mucosal m.
    infiltrative m.
    invasive m.
    irregular m.
    normal tissue m.
    sclerotic m.

mar·gin *(continued)*
    spiculated m.
    surgical m.
    tumor m.

mar·gi·na·tion

mark·er
    activation m.
    biochemical m.
    biologic m.
    cell-surface m.
    chromosomal m.
    chromosome m.
    clonal m.
    cytogenetic m.
    disease-specific m.
    enzyme m.
    epithelial m.
    genetic m.
    Ig m.
    immunohistochemical m.
    morphologic m.
    serologic m.
    serum m.
    tumor m.

Ma·ro·teaux
    M.-Lamy syndrome

Mar·ri·ott
    Levy, Rowntree, and M's
      method

mar·row
    bone m.
    CD6-depleted allogenic
      bone m.
    CD6-depleted bone m.
    depressed m.
    megaloblastic bone m.
    purged autologous m.

mar·row-de·rived

mas·chal·on·cus

mass
    mediastinal m.
    pelvic m.
    soft tissue m.
    umbilical m.

Mas·son
    Fontana-M. stain

mas·tec·to·my
    Auchincloss modified radi-
      cal m.
    extended radical m.
    Halsted m.
    Meyer m.
    modified radical m.
    partial m.
    radical m.
    segmental m.
    simple m.
    subcutaneous m.
    total m.

mas·to·cy·to·sis

match·ing
    ABO m.
    cross m.
    HLA m.

ma·te·ri·al
    cross-reacting m. (CRM)
    cross-reaction m.

ma·trix *pl.* ma·tri·ces
    bone m.

Mat·sue
    PGK-M.

Mat·u·lane

Maun·sell
    M.-Weir operation

May
    M.-Grünwald stain
    M.-Hegglin anomaly

May·er
    M's hematoxylin solution

Ma·yo
    St. Anne-M. classification
    (for astrocytomas)

may·tan·sine

M-BACOD
  methotrexate, bleomycin, doxorubicin, cyclophosphamide, vincristine, dexamethasone

MB-02 (erythroleukemia) cell line

MB-03 (megakaryoblastic) cell line

mbr
  major breakpoint region

MC
  mixed-cellularity Hodgkin's disease

MC 540
  merocyanine 540

MCC
  mutated in colorectal cancer

MCH
  mean corpuscular hemoglobin

MCHC
  mean corpuscular hemoglobin concentration

M-CHOP
  methotrexate, cyclophosphamide, doxorubicin, vincristine, and prednisone

MCOP
  methotrexate, cyclophosphamide, vincristine, prednisone, and leucovorin

MCR
  mononuclear cell reaction

mcr
  minor cluster region

M-CSF
  macrophage colony-stimulating factor

MCV
  mean corpuscular volume

M.D. An·der·son Hos·pi·tal stag·ing (for melanoma)

MDR
  multidrug resistance

MDR (multidrug resistance) gene

MDS
  myelodysplasia

meCCNU
  semustine

MeCCNU
  semustine

MeCcnu
  semustine

mech·lor·eth·amine
  m. hydrochloride

me·clo·fen·am·ate so·di·um

me·co·bal·amine

me·di·as·ti·nos·co·py

me·di·as·ti·num *pl.* **me·di·as·ti·na**
  anterior m.
  middle m.
  posterior m.

me·di·a·tor

Med·i·cal In·ter·nal Ra·di·a·tion Dose

Med·i·cal Re·search Coun·cil of Great Brit·ain

med·i·cine
  nuclear m.

Med·i·port

Med·i·ter·ra·ne·an ane·mia

Med·i·ter·ra·ne·an dis·ease

Med·i·ter·ra·nean lym·pho·ma

me·di·um *pl.* me·dia, me·di·ums
    conditioned m.

Med·ra·lone

Med·rol

med·roxy·pro·ges·te·rone
    m. acetate

Med·tron·ic Syn·chro·med In·fu·sion Sys·tem

me·dul·lo·blas·to·ma

me·dul·lo·epi·the·li·o·ma

me·dul·lo·su·pra·re·no·ma

MEG
    megestrol acetate

Meg
    megestrol acetate

Me·gace

mega·karyo·blast

mega·karyo·blas·tic

mega·karyo·cyte

mega·karyo·cyt·ic

mega·karyo·cy·to·poi·e·sis

mega·karyo·cy·to·sis

meg·a·lo·blast
    m. of Sabin

meg·a·lo·blas·toid

meg·a·lo·caryo·cyte

meg·a·lo·cyte

meg·a·lo·cy·to·sis

meg·a·lo·karyo·cyte

Meg-CSF
    megakaryocytic colony-stimulating factor

me·ges·trol ac·e·tate

Meigs
    M. syndrome

mel·a·ne·mia

mel·a·no·ac·an·tho·ma

mel·a·no·a·melo·blas·to·ma

mel·a·no·blas·to·ma

mel·a·no·car·ci·no·ma

mel·a·no·cyte

mel·a·no·cy·to·ma

mel·a·no·ma
    acral-lentiginous m.
    amelanotic m.
    anorectal m.
    m. of choroid
    choroidal m.
    ciliary body m.
    m. of ciliary body
    m. of conjunctiva
    cutaneous m.
    extraocular m.
    m. of eyelid
    familial m.
    familial atypical multiple mole m.
    intraocular m.
    iridal m.
    iris m.
    lentigo maligna m.
    malignant m. of esophagus
    malignant m. of vulva
    metastatic m.
    mixed uveal m.
    mucosal lentiginous m.
    nodular m.
    ocular m.
    primary m.
    m. in situ
    spindle cell m.
    subungual m.
    superficial spreading m.
    uveal m.
    vaginal m.
    vulvar m.

mel·a·no·ma·to·sis

mel·a·no·ma·tous

mel·a·no·phage

mel·a·no·sis
    circumscribed precancer-
        ous m. of Dubreuilh

me·lon·cus

mel·pha·lan

mem·brane
    basement m.
    erythrocyte m.
    platelet m.
    platelet demarcation m.

Me·mo·ri·al Sloan-Ket·ter·
    ing Can·cer Cen·ter

MEN
    multiple endocrine neopla-
        sia

MEN I
    multiple endocrine neopla-
        sia, type I

MEN IIa
    multiple endocrine neopla-
        sia, type IIa

MEN IIb
    multiple endocrine neopla-
        sia, type IIb

men·a·di·ol

Men·est

me·nin·gi·o·ma
    angioblastic m.
    clivus m.
    olfactory groove m.
    parasagittal m.
    post-radiation m.
    sphenoid ridge m.
    tuberculum sellae m.

me·nin·gi·o·ma·to·sis

men·in·gi·tis *pl.* men·in·git·
    i·des

men·in·gi·tis *(continued)*
    m. carcinomatosa
    chemical-induced m.

me·nin·go·blas·to·ma

me·nin·go·fi·bro·blas·to·ma

me·nin·go·ma

me·nin·go·the·li·o·ma

me·nis·co·cyte

me·nis·co·cy·to·sis

me·no·ga·ril

Meph·y·ton

Me·pro·lone

MER
    methanol extraction resi-
        due of bacille Calmette-
        Guérin

2-mer·cap·to·eth·ane sul·fate

mer·cap·to·pu·rine

6-mer·cap·to·pur·ine

Mer·kel
    M. cell tumor

mero·cy·a·nine 540 (MC 540)

MES-2
    mesna

mes·en·chy·mo·ma
    benign m.
    malignant m.

mes·na

MES·NEX

meso·cy·to·ma

meso·derm

meso·der·mal

meso·gli·o·ma

meso·hy·lo·ma

meso·ne·phro·ma

meso·the·li·o·ma
  benign m.
  malignant m.
  peritoneal m.
  pleural m.
  tunica vaginalis m.

mes·sen·ger
  first m.
  second m.
  third m.

me·tach·ro·nous

meta·gen·ic

meta·glob·u·lin

meta·he·mo·glo·bin

meta·io·do·ben·zyl·gua·ni·dine

met·al·lo·pro·tein·ase

meta·mor·pho·sis
  platelet m.
  structural m.
  viscous m.

meta·my·elo·cyte

Me·tan·dren

meta·pla·sia
  myeloid m.
  myeloid m., agnogenic
  squamous m.

meta·ru·bri·cyte

me·tas·ta·sis *pl.* me·tas·ta·ses
  adrenal m.
  distant m.
  epidural m.
  hematogenous m.
  hepatic m.
  implantation m.
  intramedullary m.
  leptomeningeal m.
  liver m.
  local m.
  nodal m.

me·tas·ta·sis *(continued)*
  osseous m.
  pulmonary m.
  regional m.
  skeletal m.
  skip m.
  spinal m.
  spinal cord m.
  synchronous m.

me·tas·ta·size

meta·stat·ic

meta·throm·bin

meta·typ·ic

meta·typ·i·cal

meth·a·nol
  absolute m.

meth·di·la·zine

met·hem·al·bu·min

met·hem·al·bu·min·emia

met·he·mo·glo·bin

met·he·mo·glo·bin·emia

met·he·mo·glo·bin·emic

meth·od
  absorption m.
  acid hematin m.
  Baumgartner perfusion m.
  Duke's m.
  Fahraeus m.
  Fichera's m.
  Folin and Wu's m.
  Howell's m.
  Ivy's m.
  Levy m.
  Levy, Rowntree, and Mar-
    riott's m.
  Marriott's m.
  Nikiforoff's m.
  Price-Jones m.
  Rowntree m.
  Sahli's m.
  Simonton m.

meth·od *(continued)*
    von Clauss m.
    Wallhauser and White-
        head's m.
    Westergren m.
    Wintrobe m.
    Wintrobe and Landsberg's
        m.

meth·od·ol·o·gy
    Roche-Wainer-Thissen m.

meth·o·trex·ate
    high-dose m.
    standard-dose m.

me·thox·sa·len

5-me·thoxy·psor·a·len

8-me·thoxy·psor·a·len

meth·yl·a·tion
    DNA m.

meth·yl·az·oxy·meth·a·nol

methylCCNU

3-meth·yl·cho·lan·threne

meth·y·lene
    m. chloride

4,4′-meth·y·lene *bis*(2-chlo·
    ro·an·i·line)

meth·y·lene tet·ra·hy·dro·
    fo·late

meth·yl·er·go·no·vine

meth·yl·for·ma·mide

methyl-GAG

meth·yl·gly·ox·al *bis* gua·
    nyl·hy·dra·zone (MGBG)

([¹¹C]methyl)-L-me·thi·o·nine

N-meth·yl-*n*-ni·tro·so·guan·
    i·dine

N-meth·yl-*n*-ni·tro·so·urea

meth·yl·pred·nis·o·lone

meth·yl·tes·tos·ter·one

meth·yl·tet·ra·hy·dro·fo·
    late

meth·yl·xan·thine

met·o·clo·pra·mide

met·o·prine

ME·TRO
    metronidazole

Me·tro

Metro
    metronidazole

me·tro·car·ci·no·ma

me·tro·fi·bro·ma

me·tro·ni·da·zole

met·ure·de·pa

MeV
    million electron volts

Mev·a·cor

Mev·a·tron

Mex·ate

Mey·er·hof
    Embden-M. pathway

MG-63 (osteosarcoma) cell line

MGBG
    methylglyoxal *bis* guanyl-
        hydrazone

MGUS
    monoclonal gammopathy
        of undetermined signifi-
        cance

MHC
    major histocompatibility
        complex

Mi-Acid

MIBG
    metaiodobenzylguanidine

Mi·che·li
  Marchiafava-M. disease
  Marchiafava-M. syndrome

mi·cro·ad·e·no·ma

mi·cro·aero·to·nom·e·ter

mi·cro·ag·gre·gate

mi·cro·an·gi·op·a·thy
  thrombotic m.

mi·cro·blast

mi·cro·cal·ci·fi·ca·tion

mi·cro·cyst

mi·cro·cyte

mi·cro·cy·the·mia

mi·cro·cy·to·sis

mi·cro·drep·a·no·cyt·ic

mi·cro·drep·a·no·cy·to·sis

mi·cro·en·cap·su·la·tion

mi·cro·eryth·ro·cyte

mi·cro·gli·o·ma

mi·cro·gli·o·ma·to·sis

mi·cro·glob·u·lin

β₂-mi·cro·glob·u·lin

mi·cro·he·ma·to·crit

mi·cro·in·fu·ser
  Abbott-Parker LifeCare
  1500 Ambulatory M.

mi·cro·in·va·sion

mi·cro·in·va·sive

Micro-K

mi·cro·leu·ko·blast

mi·cro·lym·phoido·cyte

mi·cro·mega·karyo·cyte

mi·cro·me·tas·ta·sis

mi·cro·meta·stat·ic

mi·cro·nor·mo·blast

mi·cro·pap·il·lary

mi·cro·phage

mi·cro·phago·cyte

mi·cro·pro·lac·ti·no·ma

mi·cro·pump
  Parker M.

mi·cro·re·frac·tom·e·ter
  immunofluorescence m.

mi·cro·sphere
  biodegradable starch m.
  starch m.

mi·cro·sphe·ro·cyte

mi·cro·sphe·ro·cy·to·sis

mi·cro·ves·i·cle
  platelet-derived m.

mi·cro·vis·co·sim·e·ter

mi·cro·wave

mid·gut

MIF
  macrophage-inhibiting fac-
    tor
  migration inhibiting factor

mi·gra·tion
  cell m.
  m. of leukocytes

milk
  cancer m.

MIME
  methyl GAG, ifosfamide,
    methotrexate, and etopo-
    side

mini·man·tle

mini·sat·el·lite

Min·i·tec

Min·kow·ski
  M.-Chauffard syndrome

mi·nog·a·ril

Mi·not
    M.-von Willebrand syn-
        drome

Min·tox Plus

MIP
    macrophage inflammatory
        protein

MISO
    misonidazole

Miso
    misonidazole

mi·so·nid·a·zole

Mith·ra·cin

mith·ra·my·cin

mi·to·car·cin

mi·to·cro·min

mi·to·gen
    pokeweed m.

mi·to·gua·zone

mi·to·lac·tol

mi·to·mal·cin

mi·to·my·cin
    m. C

mi·to·sis *pl.* mi·to·ses

mi·to·sper

mi·to·tane

mi·tot·ic

mi·to·xan·trone

MiV gly·co·phor·in

mixed-line·age

M3 leu·ke·mia

M1 leu·ke·mia cell

MMC C
    mitomycin C

Mmc C
    mitomycin C

MMMT
    malignant mixed mesoder-
        mal tumor

M20 (myelomonocytic) cell line

MNNG
    N-methyl-*n*-nitrosoguani-
        dine

MNU
    N-methyl-*n*-nitrosourea

MO7 (myeloid leukemia) cell
    line

MoAb
    monoclonal antibody

MOB
    mitomycin C, vincristine,
        and bleomycin sulfate

Mo·ben·ol

mo·bil·fer·rin

MOCA
    methotrexate, vincristine,
        cyclophosphamide, and
        doxorubicin

mod·el
    Berenblum m. of carcino-
        genesis
    Goldie-Coldman m.

mod·i·fi·ca·tion
    dose m.
    tiol m.

mod·i·fi·er
    biologic response m.
    biological response m.

Mod·ras·tane

mod·u·la·tion
    biochemical m.

MO7E (myeloblast) cell line

MOF
> semustine, vincristine, and
> 5-fluorouracil

Mohs
> M. chemosurgery

mole
> hydatidiform m.
> invasive m.
> malignant m.
> metastasizing m.

mol·e·cule
> cell adhesion m.
> cytoadhesion m.
> endothelial cell adhesion
> m.-1 (ELAM-1)
> homing-associated adhe-
> sion m. (H-CAm)
> intracellular adhesion m.
> (ICAM)
> intracellular adhesion m.-
> 1 (ICAM-1)
> leukocyte adhesion m.
> (LAM)
> leukocyte adhesion m.-1
> (LAM-1)
> leukocyte-endothelial cell
> adhesion m.-1 (LECAM-
> 1)
> LFA-1 adhesion m.
> LFA-3 adhesion m.
> neural cell adhesion m.
> (NCAM-1)
> platelet–endothelial cell
> adhesion m.-1 (PECAM-
> 1)
> vascular cell adhesion m.-
> 1 (VCAM-1)

mol gene

mono·blast

mono·blas·tic

mono·blas·to·ma

mono·clo·nal

mono·clo·nal·i·ty

mono·cyte
> endothelium-derived m.
> (EDM)

mono·cyt·ic

mono·cy·toid

mono·cy·to·pe·nia

mono·cy·to·poi·e·sis

mono·cy·to·sis

mono·der·mo·ma

mono·gen

mono·kine

mono·mer
> fibrin m.

mono·mor·phic

mono·nu·cle·o·sis
> cytomegalovirus m.
> infectious m.

mono·pe·nia

mono·phy·le·tism

mono·phy·le·tist

mono·poi·e·sis

mono·so·my
> m. 7

mono·va·lent

MOPLACE
> cyclophosphamide, etopo-
> side, prednisone, metho-
> trexate, cytarabine, and
> vincristine

MOPP
> mechlorethamine, vincris-
> tine, procarbazine, and
> prednisone

MOPP/ABV
> mechlorethamine hydro-
> chloride, vincristine, pro-
> carbazine, prednisone,

MOPP/ABV *(continued)*
    doxorubicin, bleomycin,
    and vinblastine

MOPP/ABVD
    mechlorethamine hydro-
    chloride, vincristine, pro-
    carbazine, prednisone,
    doxorubicin, bleomycin,
    vinblastine, and dacarba-
    zine

MOPP-re·sis·tant

mor·pho·log·ic

mor·phol·o·gy
    cell m.

mo·sa·i·cism

Mos·ler
    M's sign

Moss
    M. classification

Mosse
    M's syndrome

Mott
    M. bodies
    M. cell

MP
    6-mercaptopurine

M & P
    melphalan and prednisone

6-MP
    6-mercaptopurine

Mp
    6-mercaptopurine

6-Mp
    6-mercaptopurine

MPA
    mantle-paraaortic-splenic
    (irradiation)

MPAS
    mantle-paraaortic-splenic
    (irradiation)

MPI Py·ro·phos·phate

MPI Xe·non Xe 133 Gas

MPO (myeloperoxidase) de·fi·
    cien·cy

M pro·tein

M-2 pro·to·col

MPS
    mononuclear phagocyte
    system

MR
    medical report

MRC
    Medical Research Council
    of Great Britain

MRI
    magnetic resonance imag-
    ing

MSKCC
    Memorial Sloan-Kettering
    Cancer Center

MSKCC regimen
    modified MSKCC r.

99mTc-MDP
    technetium Tc-99m meth-
    ylene diphosphonate

MTD
    maximally tolerated dose

MTX
    methotrexate

Mtx
    methotrexate

MTX-CHOP
    methotrexate, cyclophos-
    phamide, doxorubicin,
    vincristine, and predni-
    sone

mu·cil·loid
    psyllium hydrophilic m.

mu·cin
    epithelial m.

mu·cin-neg·a·tive

mu·ci·nous

mu·cin-pos·i·tive

mu·co·ep·i·der·moid

mu·co·sa
    buccal m.
    gastrointestinal m.

mu·co·si·tis
    m. necroticans agranulocy-
    tica

Muir
    M. syndrome

Mül·ler
    blood dust (of M.)

mül·le·ri·a·no·ma

mül·le·ri·an tu·mor

mul·ti·cen·tric

multi-CSF
    multicolony-stimulating
    factor (interleukin 3)

mul·ti·drug

mul·ti·fo·cal

Mul·ti-in·sti·tu·tion·al Os·
teo·sar·co·ma Stu·dy

mul·ti·mer
    vWF (von Willebrand fac-
    tor) m.

mul·ti·mer·in

mul·ti·mer·iza·tion

mul·ti·nu·cle·at·ed

Mul·ti·pax

mul·ti·va·lent

mul·ti·ve·sic·u·lar

MUO
    metastasis of unknown or-
    igin

MUO syn·drome

Mur·chi·son
    M.-Sanderson syndrome

mu·ro·mon·ab-CD3

Mur·phy
    M. cycle A

Mus·cu·lo·skel·e·tal Tu·mor
So·ci·ety

MUST
    mechlorethamine hydro-
    chloride (Mustargen)

Must
    mechlorethamine hydro-
    chloride (Mustargen)

mus·tard
    m. gas
    nitrogen m.
    phenylalanine m.
    L-phenylalamine m.
    sulfur m.
    uracil m.

Mus·tar·gen

mu·ta·gen

mu·ta·gen·e·sis
    insertional m.

mu·ta·gen·ic

mu·ta·ge·nic·i·ty

Mu·ta·my·cin

mu·tant

mu·ta·tion
    frameshift m.
    GAA→TAA m.
    normoblastosis m.
    point m.
    scat m.

mu·ta·tion·al

MVAC
    methotrexate, vinblastine, doxorubicin, and cisplatin

M-VAC
    methotrexate, vinblastine, doxorubicin, and cisplatin

MVPP
    mechlorethamine, vinblastine, procarbazine, prednisone

my·as·the·nia
    m. gravis

My·ce·lex

my·co·sis
    m. fungoides
    m. fungoides d'emblée

my·el·emia

my·elo·blast

my·elo·blas·te·mia

my·elo·blas·tic

my·elo·blas·to·ma

my·elo·blas·to·ma·to·sis

my·elo·blas·to·sis

my·elo·cyte

my·elo·cy·the·mia

my·elo·cyt·ic

my·elo·cy·to·ma

my·elo·cy·to·sis

my·elo·dys·pla·sia

my·elo·dys·plas·tic

my·elo·fi·bro·sis
    acute m.
    idiopathic m.
    malignant m.
    primary m.
    secondary m.

my·elo·gen·ic

my·elog·e·nous

my·elo·gone

my·elo·gon·ic

my·elo·go·ni·um

my·elo·gram

my·elog·ra·phy

my·eloid

my·elo·ken·tric

my·elo·li·po·ma

my·elo·ma
    endothelial m.
    giant cell m.
    IgA m.
    IgG m.
    indolent m.
    localized m.
    multiple m.
    plasma cell m.
    smoldering m.
    solitary m.

my·elo·ma·toid

my·elo·ma·to·sis

my·elo·mono·cyt·ic

my·elom·y·ces

my·elop·a·thy
    radiation m.

my·e·lo·per·ox·i·dase (MPO)

my·e·lo·per·ox·i·dase (MPO) de·fi·cien·cy

my·elo·phthi·sis

my·elo·plaque

my·elo·plast

my·elo·plax

my·elo·poi·e·sis

my·elo·pro·lif·er·a·tion

my·elo·pro·lif·er·a·tive

my·elo·sar·co·ma

my·elo·sar·co·ma·to·sis

my·elo·scle·ro·sis

my·el·o·sis
    aleukemic m.
    chronic megakaryocytic-
      granulocytic m.
    chronic nonleukemic m.
    erythremic m.
    megakaryocytic m.
    nonleukemic m.

my·elo·sup·pres·sion
    chemotherapy-induced m.
    cytarabine-induced m.
    5-fluorouracil–induced m.

my·elo·sup·pres·sive

my·elo·tox·ic

my·elo·tox·ic·i·ty

My·gel

Myhre
    Ruvalcaba-M.-Smith syn-
      drome

Myi·dil

Myl·er·an

My·li·con

myo·blas·to·ma
    granular cell m.

myo·blas·to·my·o·ma

myo·cy·to·ma

myo·epi·the·li·o·ma

myo·fi·bro·ma

myo·li·po·ma

my·o·ma *pl.* my·o·mas, my·
  o·ma·ta
    ball m.
    m. sarcomatodes
    m. striocellulare
    m. telangiectodes

my·o·ma·gen·e·sis

my·o·ma·ta

my·o·ma·to·sis

my·o·ma·tous

myo·sar·co·ma

myo·schwan·no·ma

my·os·te·o·ma

myx·ad·e·no·ma

myxo·ad·e·no·ma

myxo·blas·to·ma

myxo·chon·dro·fi·bro·sar·co·
  ma

myxo·chon·dro·ma

myxo·chon·dro·sar·co·ma

myxo·cys·to·ma

myxo·en·chon·dro·ma

myxo·en·do·the·li·o·ma

myxo·fi·bro·ma

myxo·fi·bro·sar·co·ma

myxo·gli·o·ma

myxo·in·o·ma

myxo·li·po·ma

myx·o·ma *pl.* myx·o·mas,
  myx·o·ma·ta
    cystic m.
    enchondromatous m.
    erectile m.
    m. fibrosum
    lipomatous m.
    m. sarcomatosum
    vascular m.

myx·o·ma·to·sis

myx·o·ma·tous

myxo·my·o·ma

myxo·pap·il·lo·ma

myxo·sar·co·ma

myxo·sar·co·ma·tous

MZ (monozygotic) twin·ning

NAD
    neutrophil actin dysfunction
    nucleoside adenine phosphate

Na·di
    N. reaction

Nae·ge·li
    N. leukemia
    microblast of N.

naf·ox·i·dine hy·dro·chlo·ride

Nak-a plate·let

nal·i·dix·ic acid

Nan·dro·bol·ic

nan·dro·lone
    n. decanoate
    n. phenpropionate

naph·thol
    n. AS-MX phosphate
    n. AS phosphate

2-naph·thyl·amine

naph·thyl·para·ro·san·i·line

na·so·phar·ynx

Na·tion·al Blad·der Can·cer Col·lab·o·ra·tive Group A

Na·tion·al Can·cer In·sti·tute

Na·tion·al Pro·stat·ic Can·cer Pro·ject

Na·tion·al Sur·gi·cal Ad·ju·vant Breast and Bow·el Pro·ject

Na·tion·al Wilms' Tu·mor Stu·dy Group

Na·tu·lan

nau·sea

NB4 cell line

NBCCGA
    National Bladder Cancer Collaborative Group A

NCAM-1
    neural cell adhesion molecule-1

NCCTG
    North Central Cancer Treatment Group

NCI
    National Cancer Institute

5'-ND
    5'-nucleotidase

ndHPFH
    nondeletional hereditary persistence of fetal hemoglobin

neb·u·lar·ine

ne·cro·sis *pl.* ne·cro·ses
    n. of bone marrow
    coagulation n.
    pseudopalisading n.
    radiation n.
    tumor n.

NED
    no evidence of disease

nee·dle
    butterfly n.
    Huber n.
    scalp-vein n.

nef gene

Neis·ser
    N.-Wechsberg phenomenon

Neis·se·ria
    N. meningitidis

Neis·se·ria (continued)
  N. subflava

Né·la·ton
  N's tumor

neo·ad·ju·vant

neo·an·ti·gen

neo·car·zi·no·sta·tin

Neo-Co·de·ma

neo·cy·to·sis

neo·den·si·ty

Neo-Dur·a·bol·ic

Neo-Es·trone

neo gene

neo·my·cin

neo·na·tal

neo·pla·sia
  cervical intraepithelial n.
  colonic n.
  gestational trophoblastic
    n.
  Hürthle cell n.
  multiple endocrine n.
    (MEN)
  trophoblastic n.
  vaginal intraepithelial n.

neo·plasm
  abdominal n.
  CNS n.
  histoid n.
  low-grade n.
  lymphoid n.
  lymphoproliferative blood
    cell n.
  neuroendocrine n.
  organoid n.
  plasma cell n.
  primary n.
  second n.
  secondary n.

neo·plas·tic

ne·o·plas·ti·gen·ic

ne·op·ter·in

Neo·sar

Neo·scan

neph·rad·e·no·ma

ne·phrec·to·my
  radical n.

neph·ro·blas·to·ma

neph·ro·blas·to·ma·to·sis

ne·phro·ma
  congenital mesoblastic n.
  embryonal n.
  mesoblastic n.

neph·ron·cus

ne·phrop·a·thy
  urate n.
  uric acid n.

ne·phros·to·my
  percutaneous n.

neph·ro·tox·ic

neph·ro·tox·ic·i·ty

neph·ro·tox·in

Nep·ta·zane

nerve
  cranial n's

ne·sid·io·blas·to·ma

nest
  cancer n's
  squamous n.

Neu·po·gen

neur·ad·e·nol·y·sis

neu·ri·lem·mo·ma

neu·ri·no·ma

neu·ro·as·tro·cy·to·ma

neu·ro·blas·to·ma
  olfactory n.

neu·ro·cy·to·ma

neu·ro·epi·the·li·o·ma

neu·ro·fi·bro·ma

neu·ro·fi·bro·ma·to·sis

neu·ro·fi·bro·sar·co·ma

neu·ro·glio·cy·to·ma

neu·ro·gli·o·ma

neu·ro·gli·o·ma·to·sis

neu·ro·gli·o·sis

neu·ro·imag·ing

neu·ro·ma
    malignant n.

neu·ro-on·co·log·ic

neu·ro-on·col·o·gy

neu·ro·ra·di·ol·o·gy

neu·ro·sar·co·ma

neu·ro·spon·gi·o·ma

neu·ro·tox·ic·i·ty

Neu·tra-Phos

neu·tro·cyte

neu·tro·cy·to·pe·nia

neu·tro·cy·to·sis

neu·tro·pe·nia
    autoimmune n. of infancy
    chronic benign n. of child-
      hood
    chronic hypoplastic n.
    congenital n.
    cyclic n.
    familial benign chronic n.
    hypersplenic n.
    idiopathic n.
    Kostmann n.
    malignant n.
    neonatal n., transitory
    periodic n.
    peripheral n.

neu·tro·pe·nia *(continued)*
    primary splenic n.

neu·tro·phil
    filamented n.
    giant n.
    juvenile n.
    nonfilamented n.
    rod n.
    stab n.

neu·tro·phil·ia

neu·tro·tax·is

ne·vus *pl.* ne·vi
    blue n.
    congenital n.
    dysplastic n.
    junctional n.
    sebaceous n.
    n. sebaceus
    n. sebaceus of Jadassohn

Nez·e·lof
    N. syndrome

NF-*jun* gene

NGF
    nerve growth factor

NH
    nodular histiocytic lym-
      phoma

NHL
    nodular histiocytic lym-
      phoma
    non-Hodgkin's lymphoma

Nia-Bid

Ni·ac

Ni·a·cels

ni·a·cin

ni·a·cin·amide

nick·el

Nico-400

Nic·o·bid

Nic·o·lar

Nic·o·tin·ex Elix·ir

NIH 3T3 (fibroblast) cell line

Ni·ki·fo·roff
    N's method

nip·ple
    Paget's disease of n.

ni·tric ox·ide syn·thase

ni·trite

ni·tro·blue tet·ra·zo·li·um

ni·tro·gen
    n. mustards
    nonprotein n.
    rest n.

ni·tro·im·id·az·ole

ni·tro·prus·side

N-ni·tros·amide

ni·tros·amine

ni·tro·so·al·kyl·car·ba·mate

ni·tro·so(al·kyl)guan·i·dine

ni·tro·so(al·kyl)urea

N-ni·tro·so·di·eth·yl·amine

N-ni·tro·so·di·meth·yl·
    amine

N-ni·tro·so·meth·yl·urea

ni·tro·so·urea
    n. S 10036

ni·tro·so·ure·thane

ni·za·ti·dine

Niz·oral

NK
    natural killer (cells)

NKM-1 (myeloid) cell line

NM
    nodular melanoma

NM *(continued)*
    nodular mixed histiocytic-
    lymphocytic lymphoma

NML
    nodular mixed histiocytic-
    lymphocytic lymphoma

N-*myc* on·co·gene

no·co·da·zole

no·dal

node
    axillary n.
    axillary lymph n's
    cervical lymph n's
    Ewald's n.
    groin n.
    ilioinguinal lymph n's
    inguinal n.
    inguinal lymph n's
    internal mammary lymph
       n's
    lower cervical lymph n's
    lymph n.
    mediastinal lymph n's
    neck n's
    parotid lymph n's
    Rotter's n's
    sentinel n.
    signal n.
    supraclavicular lymph n's
    Troisier's n.
    Virchow's n.
    upper cervical lymph n's

node-neg·a·tive

node-pos·i·tive
    pulmonary n's
    Sister Joseph's n.
    solitary pulmonary n.
    tumor n.

nod·u·lar

nod·ule

no·gal·a·my·cin

Nola·hist

Nol·va·dex

Nol·va·dex-D

no·men·cla·ture
    CD n.

NOMO-1 cell line

non·cleaved

non·on·co·gen·ic

non·poly·po·sis

non·re·sponse

non·se·cre·tor

non·sem·i·no·ma·tous

NOP
    mitoxantrone, vincristine,
        and prednisolone

nor·epi·neph·rine

nor·mo·blast
    acidophilic n.
    basophilic n.
    early n.
    eosinophilic n.
    intermediate n.
    late n.
    orthochromatic n.
    oxyphilic n.
    polychromatic n.

nor·mo·blas·tic

nor·mo·blas·to·sis

nor·mo·cal·ce·mia

nor·mo·cal·ce·mic

nor·mo·chro·ma·sia

nor·mo·chro·mia

nor·mo·chro·mic

nor·mo·cyte

nor·mo·cyt·ic

nor·mo·cy·to·sis

nor·mo·eryth·ro·cyte

nor·mo-or·tho·cy·to·sis

nor·mo·skeo·cy·to·sis

nor·mo·vo·le·mia

nor·mo·vo·le·mic

Nor·port

Nor·port-LS

Nor·port-SP

Nor-Pred T.B.A.

Nor·ris
    N. corpuscles

North Cen·tral Can·cer Treat·
    ment Group

Northern blot

Northern blot analysis

Nor·ton
    N.-Simon hypothesis

no·to·chor·do·ma

No·van·trone

No·vo·bu·ta·mide

No·vo·ci·me·tine

No·vo·fi·brate

No·vo·hy·droxy·zin

No·vo·lente-K

No·vo·py·ra·zone

No·vo·sem·ide

NOVP
    mitoxantrone, vincristine,
    vinblastine, and predni-
    sone

NPCP
    National Prostatic Cancer
    Project

NPDL
    nodular, poorly differen-
    tiated lymphocytic lym-
    phoma

NPS
National Polyp Study

N-*ras* on·co·gene

NRD
negative regulatory do-
main

NSABP
National Surgical Adju-
vant Breast and Bowel
Project

NSCLC
non–small cell lung cancer

NSD
nominal single dose

nu·cle·ase
S1 n.

nu·cle·oid

nu·cle·o·lus *pl.* nu·cle·o·li
inclusionlike n.

nu·cleo·phago·cy·to·sis

nu·cleo·plasm

nu·cleo·side
n. adenine diphosphate
(NAD)
tricyclic n. phosphate

nu·cleo·side phos·phate
tricyclic n.p.

5′-nu·cle·o·ti·dase

nu·cleo·tide
adenine n.

nu·cle·us *pl.* nu·clei
drumstick n.

NWDL
nodular well-differentiated
lymphocytic lymphoma

NWTSG
National Wilms' Tumor
Study Group

nys·ta·tin

O
    vincristine (Oncovin)

OAF
    osteoclast activating factor

Oak·ley
    O.-Fulthorpe technique
    O.-Fulthorpe test

OAP
    vincristine, cytarabine,
      and prednisone

ob·struc·tion
    biliary o.

OC-2008 (ovarian carcinoma)
    cell line
    catheter o.

oc·ton·ic acid

oc·treo·tide
    o. acetate

Ohn·gren
    O's line

OH-urea
    hydroxyurea

oil
    ethiodized o.
    fish o.

OK-432

Old·field
    O's syndrome

ol·i·ge·mia

ol·i·ge·mic

ol·i·go 2′,5′-aden·yl·ate syn·
  thase

ol·i·go·as·tro·cy·to·ma
    mixed o.

ol·i·go·chro·ma·sia

ol·i·go·chro·me·mia

ol·i·go·clo·nal

ol·i·go·cy·the·mia

ol·i·go·cy·them·ic

ol·i·go·cy·to·sis

ol·i·go·den·dro·blas·to·ma

ol·i·go·den·dro·gli·al

ol·i·go·den·dro·gli·o·ma

ol·i·go·den·dro·ma

ol·i·go·he·mia

ol·i·go·nu·cle·o·tide
    anti-sense o.

ol·i·go·sac·cha·ride

ome·pra·zole

Om·ma·ya
    O. reservoir

om·pha·lo·ma

om·pha·lon·cus

ONC
    over-the-needle catheter

ONCOCIN sys·tem

on·co·cyte

on·co·cyt·ic

on·co·cy·to·ma

on·co·fe·tal

on·co·gene
    abl o.
    c-o.
    c-*erb* B₂ o.
    c-*fgr* o.
    c-*jun* o.
    c-*kit* o.
    c-*myb* o.
    c-*myc* o.
    c-*ras* o.

on·co·gene *(continued)*
    HER-2/*neu* o.
    H-*ras* o.
    K-*ras* o.
    met o.
    neu o.
    N-*myc* o.
    N-*ras* o.
    ras o.
    v-o.

on·co·gen·e·sis

on·co·ge·net·ic

on·co·gen·ic

on·co·ge·nic·i·ty

on·cog·e·nous

on·col·o·gy
    gynecologic o.
    medical o.
    radiation o.
    surgical o.

on·col·y·sate
    viral o.

on·col·y·sis

on·co·lyt·ic

on·co·ma

on·co·Rad OV103

on·co·sis

on·co·ther·a·py

on·co·thlip·sis

on·co·trop·ic

On·co·vin

On·co·vor·in

on·dan·e·tron hy·dro·chlo·ride

on·dan·se·tron

on·tog·e·ny

ooph·o·rec·to·my
    prophylactic o.

o,p′-DDD
    mitotane

OPEC
    vincristine, prednisone, etoposide, and chlorambucil

op·er·a·tion
    Black o.
    Localio o.
    Maunsell-Weir o.
    pull-through o.
    second-look o.
    Tikhor-Linberg o.
    transsacral o.
    Turnbull-Cutait o.

op·sin·og·e·nous

op·son·ic

op·so·nin

op·so·ni·za·tion

op·so·nize

op·so·no·cy·to·phag·ic

op·so·no·phil·ia

op·so·no·phil·ic

Op·ti·mine

Or·a·mide

or·ange
    o. G
    thiazole o.

Ora-Tes·tryl

or·chi·ec·to·my

or·chi·en·ceph·a·lo·ma

Or·e·ton

Or·fit

or·gan
    target o.

or·gan·i·za·tion

or·ga·no·ma

or·ga·no·plat·i·num

or·i·gin
    ectodermal o.
    endodermal o.
    mesodermal o.

Or·i·mune

Or·i·nase

or·ma·pla·tin

oro·phar·ynx

or·tho·chro·mia

or·tho·cy·to·sis

OSE
    ovarian surface epithelium

Os·ler
    O's disease
    O.-Vaquez disease

os·mo·ther·a·py

os·teo·ar·throp·a·thy
    hypertrophic pulmonary o.
    paraneoplastic o.

os·teo·blas·to·ma

os·teo·chon·dro·fi·bro·ma

os·teo·chon·dro·ma
    fibrosing o.

os·teo·chon·dro·ma·to·sis

os·teo·chon·dro·myx·o·ma

os·teo·chon·dro·phyte

os·teo·chon·dro·sar·co·ma

os·teo·clas·to·ma

os·teo·der·mia

os·teo·en·chon·dro·ma

os·teo·fi·bro·chon·dro·sar·co·ma

os·teo·fi·bro·ma

os·te·o·gen·ic

os·te·oid

os·teo·lipo·chon·dro·ma

os·teo·li·po·ma

os·te·o·ma
    cavalryman's o.
    compact o.
    o. cutis
    o. durum
    o. eburneum
    giant osteoid o.
    o. medullare
    osteoid o.
    o. sarcomatosum
    o. spongiosum

os·teo·ma·toid

os·teo·ma·to·sis

os·teo·myxo·chon·dro·ma

os·teo·ne·cro·sis

os·teo·pe·tro·sis
    autosomal recessive–lethal
      o.

os·teo·sar·co·ma
    classical o.
    mandibular o.
    maxillary o.
    parosteal o.
    periosteal o.
    small-cell o.
    telangiectatic o.

os·teo·sar·co·ma·tous

os·te·o·sis
    o. cutis

os·teo·te·lan·gi·ec·ta·sia

os·to·my

o-tol·u·i·dine

oto·tox·ic·i·ty

Ouch·ter·lo·ny
    O. technique

Ou·din
    O. technique
ova·lo·cy·tary
ovalo·cyte
ovalo·cy·to·sis
over·ex·pres·sion
over·trans·fu·sion
Ovol
Ow·ren
    O's buffer
    O's disease

ox·a·le·mia

ox·an·dro·lone

ox·i·sur·an

ox·y·gen
    hyperbaric o.

oxy·heme

oxy·he·mo·chro·mo·gen

oxy·he·mo·glo·bin

oxy·to·cin

P
    progression

PA
    pilocytic astrocytoma

PAC
    cisplatin, doxorubicin, cy-
        clophosphamide

PA6 cell

pack-year

PADGEM
    platelet activation–depen-
        dent granule–external
        membrane (protein)

Pa·get
    P's cell
    P. disease
    P's disease, extramam-
        mary
    P's disease of nipple

pag·et·oid

PAH
    polycyclic aromatic hydro-
        carbon

pain
    bone p.

pair
    base p.

Pal·ade
    Weibel-P. body

pal·ate

pal·i·sade

pal·li·a·tion

pal·li·a·tive

PAM
    melphalan

L-PAM
    melphalan

Pam
    melphalan

pan·ag·glu·tin·a·ble

pan·ag·glu·ti·na·tion

pan·ag·glu·ti·nin

Pan·coast
    P's syndrome
    P's tumor

pan·cre·as *pl.* pan·cre·a·ta
    endocrine p.
    exocrine p.

pan·cre·a·tec·to·my

pan·cre·at·i·co·du·o·de·nec·
    to·my

Pan·cre·tec 2000 pump

pan·cy·to·pe·nia
    Fanconi's p.

Pan·ec·tyl

pan·hem·a·to·pe·nia
    primary splenic p.

pan·hy·per·emia

pan·hy·po·gam·ma·glob·u·
    lin·emia

pan·my·eloid

pan·my·elo·pa·thia

pan·my·elop·a·thy

pan·my·elo·phthi·sis

Pan·or·ex

pan·to·the·nic acid

PAP
    placental alkaline phos-
        phatase

PAP *(continued)*
   placental anticoagulant
   protein

Pa·pa·nic·o·laou
   P. smear
   P. stain

pa·pil·lo·ad·e·no·cys·to·ma

pa·pil·lo·car·ci·no·ma

pap·il·lo·ma
   p. of choroid plexus
   exophytic p.
   fibroepithelial p.
   intracystic p.
   inverted p.
   inverting p.
   squamous p.
   urothelial p.
   villous p.

pap·il·lo·ma·to·sis
   diffuse p.

pap·il·lom·a·tous

pap·il·lo·ma·vi·rus
   human p.

Pap·pen·heim
   lymphoid hemoblast of P.

Pap·pen·hei·mer
   P. bodies

PAP (peroxidase-
antiperoxidase) tech·nique

Pap smear

pap·u·lo·sis
   lymphoid p.
   lymphomatoid p.
   malignant atrophic p.

para·cen·te·sis

para·crine

para·gan·gli·o·ma
   medullary p.
   nonchromaffin p.

para·gran·u·lo·ma
   nodular p.

para·he·mo·phil·ia

para·neo·plas·tic

para·ne·phro·ma

Para·pla·tin

para·pro·tein

para·pro·tein·emia

para·pso·ri·a·sis
   large plaque p.
   p. lichenoides
   p. en plaques
   poikilodermic p.
   poikilodermatous p.

para·ro·san·i·line

para·thy·roid

para·thy·roid·o·ma

para·tope

Par·ben·em

par·en·chy·ma
   p. glandulare prostatae

par·en·chy·mal

Par·ker
   Abbott-P. LifeCare 1500
      Ambulatory Microinfuser
   P. Micropump

par·os·te·al

par·ox·ys·mal

par·ti·cle
   Zimmermann's elementary
   p's

Pas·so·voy
   P. factor

patho·gen·e·sis

path·way
   alternate p.
   alternative complement p.

path·way *(continued)*
    classic p.
    classic complement p.
    coagulation p.
    common p. of coagulation
    Embden-Meyerhof p.
    extrinsic p. of coagulation
    glycolytic p.
    intrinsic p. of coagulation
    lipoxygenase p.
    properdin p.

pa·tient
    cancer p.
    high-risk p.
    poor-risk p.

pat·tern
    Regaud p.
    Schmincke p.

Pat·ter·son
    P.-Kelly syndrome

PBEI (Pre-B lymphoblast) cell line

PBL
    peripheral blood lympho-
    cyte

PBRT
    partial-brain radiotherapy

PC
    cisplatin and cyclophos-
    phamide

PC2
    procarbazine

PCNA
    proliferating cell nuclear
    antigen

PCR
    pathologically confirmed
    complete remission
    polymerase chain reaction

pCR
    pathologic complete re-
    sponse

PCV
    procarbazine, lomustine,
    and vincristine

PCVP
    procarbazine, cyclophos-
    phamide, vinblastine,
    and prednisone

PDGF
    platelet-derived growth
    factor

PDQ sys·tem

PE
    Pseudomonas exotoxin

Pearce
    Brown-P. tumor

pearl
    epidermic p's
    epithelial p's

PEB
    cisplatin, etoposide, and
    bleomycin sulfate

PECAM-1
    platelet–endothelial cell
    adhesion molecule-1

Pe·di·a·pred

Pe·di·at·ric On·col·o·gy Group

Pe·di·at·ric On·col·o·gy Group stag·ing (for neuroblastoma)

ped·i·cle
    lymphovascular p.

pe·dun·cu·lat·ed

PEG-L-as·par·a·gin·ase

Pel
    P.-Ebstein disease
    P.-Ebstein fever

Pel·ger
    P.-Huët nuclear anomaly
    pseudo–P.-Huët anomaly

pel·vis *pl.* pel·ves, pelvises

pe·nec·to·my

pen·ta·meth·yl·mel·amine

pen·tam·i·dine

Pen·ta·span

pen·ta·starch

Pen·ta·zine

pen·to·san poly·sul·fate

pen·to·sta·tin

pen·tox·i·fyl·line

pep·lo·my·cin

pep·ti·dase
 signal p.

pep·tide
 connective tissue activating p. (CTAP)
 gastrin-relasing p.
 neurogastrointestinal p's
 neutrophil activating p.
 Tac p.
 vasoactive intestinal p.
  (VIP)

Pep·tol

per·fo·ra·tion

per·fu·sion
 protein A plasma p.

peri·am·pul·lary

peri·an·gi·o·ma

peri·car·dio·cen·te·sis

peri·car·di·tis
 postirradiation p.
 radiation p.

peri·car·di·um

peri·chon·dro·ma

peri·cy·to·ma

peri·epi·the·li·o·ma

peri·os·te·al

peri·os·te·um

peri·po·le·sis

peri·the·li·o·ma

peri·to·ne·os·co·py

peri·tu·mor·al

peri·vas·cu·lar

per·kal·li·kre·in
 plasma p.

pe·rox·i·dase

per·ox·i·da·tion
 lipid p.

per·phen·a·zine

Per·san·tine

per·sist·ence
 hereditary p. of fetal hemoglobin (HPFH)
 hereditary p. of hemoglobin F

PET
 positron emission tomog-
  raphy

pe·te·chia *pl.* pe·tech·iae

Pe·ters
 P. classification (for Hodgkin's disease)

Peutz
 P.-Jeghers polyp
 P.-Jeghers syndrome

PEX
 plasma exchange

PF
 platelet factor (1–4)

PF1
 platelet factor 1

PF2
 platelet factor 2

PF3
    platelet factor 3

PF4
    platelet factor 4

PFI
    progression-free interval

PFL
    cisplatin, 5-fluorouracil,
      and leucovorin

PFX
    progression-free survival

PGK
    phosphoglycerate kinase

PGK-Mat·sue

P-gly·co·pro·tein

PGO en·zymes

P-gp
    P-glycoprotein

PgR
    progesterone receptor

PHA
    phytohemagglutinin

phago·cyt·a·ble

phago·cyte
    mononuclear p.

phago·cyt·ic

phago·cy·tin

phago·cyt·ize

phago·cy·tol·y·sis

phago·cy·to·lyt·ic

phago·cy·tose

phago·cy·to·sis
    induced p.
    spontaneous p.
    surface p.

phago·cy·tot·ic

pha·gol·y·sis

phago·ly·so·some

phago·lyt·ic

phago·some

Phar·mo·ru·bi·cin

phar·ynx

phase
    radial growth p.
    vertical growth p.

Pha·zyme

phe·nac·e·tin

Phen·a·meth

Phen·a·zine

Phen·cen-50

Phen·er·gan

phe·nin·da·mine

phe·no·bar·bi·tal

Phe·no·ject-50

phe·nol·phthal·ein

phe·nol·phthal·ein glu·cu·
    ron·ic acid

phe·nom·e·non *pl.* phe·nom·
  e·na
    Bordet-Gengou p.
    Danysz's p.
    first-set p.
    Gengou p.
    Hamburger p.
    heme-heme interaction p.
    Lewis' p.
    Neisser-Wechsberg p.
    Raynaud's p.
    second-set p.

phe·no·thi·a·zine

phe·no·type
    B-cell p.
    Bombay p.
    Dantu p.
    immunologic p.

phe·no·type *(continued)*
    Leach p.
    MDR (multidrug resis-
        tance) p.
    MiV(J.L.) p.
    null-cell p.
    senescent p.
    St[a] p.
    T-cell p.

phe·no·typ·ic

phen·oxy·ben·za·mine

phen·yl·al·a·nine
    p. mustard

phen·yl·eph·rine

phen·yl·eph·rine hy·dro·
    chlo·ride

phen·y·to·in

pheo·chro·mo·cy·to·ma
    adrenal p.

phe·re·sis

Phil·a·del·phia chromosome

phle·bot·o·my

phor·bol
    p. myristate acetate
        (PMA)

phos·pha·tase

phos·phate
    chromic p.
    polyestradiol p.

phos·pha·te·mia

phos·pha·ti·dic acid

phos·pha·ti·dic ac·id phos·
    pho·hy·dro·lase

phos·pha·ti·dyl·cho·line

phos·pha·ti·dyl·eth·a·nol·
    amine

phos·pha·ti·dyl·in·o·si·tol
    p. bisphosphate

phos·pha·ti·dyl·ser·ine

Phos·pho·col P 32

phos·pho·di·es·ter·ase

phos·pho·fruc·to·ki·nase
    muscle-type p.

phos·pho·glyc·er·ate ki·nase

phos·pho·hex·ose isom·er·ase

phos·pho·ino·si·tide

phos·pho·lip·ase

phos·pho·lip·id

phos·pho·lip·i·de·mia

phos·pho·ri·bo·syl·py·ro·
    phos·phate

phos·pho·rus
    p. 32
    radioactive p.

phos·phor·y·la·tion
    oxidative p.

Phos·pho·tec

phos·pho·tung·stic acid

pho·to·al·ler·gy
    chemotherapy-induced p.

pho·to·che·mo·ther·a·py

pho·to·co·ag·u·la·tion

pho·to·dy·nam·ic

Pho·to·fi·brin II

pho·to·met·he·mo·glo·bin

pho·to·ra·di·a·tion

pho·to·sen·si·tiv·i·ty
    chemotherapy-induced p.

pho·to·ther·a·py

pho·to·tox·ic·i·ty
    chemotherapy-induced p.

phyl·lode

phy·ma·to·rhu·sin

phy·ma·tor·rhys·in

phy·sal·i·des

phys·a·lif·er·ous

phy·sal·i·form

phy·sal·i·phore

phys·a·liph·o·rous

phys·a·lis *pl.* phys·al·i·des

phy·to·hem·ag·glu·ti·nin

phy·to·na·di·one

pi·ar·he·mia

pi·as·tri·ne·mia

Pi·az·za
     P's fluid

PICC
     percutaneously inserted
        central catheter

pic·ryl
     p. chloride

piece
     secretory p.

pig·ment
     blood p.

pi·lo·car·pine

pi·lo·cys·tic

pi·lo·cyte

pi·lo·cyt·ic

pim·e·lo·ma

pin·e·a·lo·blas·to·ma

pin·e·a·lo·cy·to·ma

pin·e·a·lo·ma
     ectopic p.

pin·eo·blas·to·ma

pin·eo·cy·to·ma

pi·o·ne·mia

pi·per·az·in·ed·i·one

pi·po·bro·man

pi·po·sul·fan

pir·ox·i·cam

Pi·to·cin

PJ
     Peutz-Jeghers syndrome

PJS
     Peutz-Jeghers syndrome

PKA
     protein kinase A

pla·kins

pla·no·cyte

plaque
     endocardial p.

Pla·que·nil

plas·ma
     antihemophilic human p.
     blood p.
     citrated p.
     normal human p.
     oxalate p.
     pooled p.
     salt p.
     true p.

plas·ma·blast

Plas·ma-CEF

plas·ma cell dis·or·der

plas·ma·cyte

plas·ma·cyt·ic

plas·ma·cy·toid

plas·ma·cy·to·ma
     extramedullary p.
     multiple p. of bone
     solitary p.
     solitary p. of bone

plas·ma·cy·to·sis

plas·mal

plas·mal·o·gen

plas·ma·phe·re·sis
  exchange p.

plas·ma·ther·a·py

plas·mat·ic

plas·mic

plas·min·o·gen
  Glu-p.
  Lys-p.

plas·mo·cyte

plas·mo·cy·to·ma

plas·mo·ma

pla·teau

plate·let
  blood p.
  giant p.
  Nak-a p.
  reticulated p.

plate·let ca·sein ki·nase

plate·let·phe·re·sis

Pla·ti·nol

plat·i·num
  p. diamminodichloride

cis-plat·i·num II

plat·i·num/Vp-16
  cisplatin and etoposide

pleo·cy·to·sis
  central nervous system p.

pleo·mor·phic

pleo·mor·phism
  nuclear p.

pleth·o·ra

ple·thor·ic

ple·thys·mog·ra·phy
  impedance p.

pleu·ra *pl.* pleu·rae

pleu·rec·to·my

pleu·rod·e·sis

pleu·ro·pneu·mo·nec·to·my

plex·us *pl.* plex·us, plex·us·es
  choroid p.
  Cruveilhier's p.

pli·ca·my·cin

Plim·mer
  P's bodies

ploi·dy
  tumor p.

PLT
  primed lymphocyte typing

plug
  hemostatic p.
  Luer-Lok p.

PMA
  phorbol myristate acetate

PMS Per·phen·a·zine

PMS Pro·chlor·per·a·zine

PMS Pro·meth·a·zine

PMS So·di·um Poly·sty·rene
  Sul·fo·nate

PMW
  pokeweed mitogen

PNET
  primitive neuroectodermal
    tumor

pneu·mo·cys·to·gram

pneu·mo·cys·tog·ra·phy

pneu·mo·nec·to·my

pneu·mo·nia
  Pneumocystis carinii p.

pneu·mo·ni·tis
  interstitial p.
  radiation p.

PNH
  paroxysmal nocturnal he-
    moglobinuria

p-ni·tro·phe·nol

PO
    L. per os (by mouth, orally)

podo·phyl·lin

podo·phyl·lo·tox·in

podo·phyl·lum

POG
    Pediatric Oncology Group

POG stag·ing (for neuroblastoma)

poi·ki·lo·blast

poi·ki·lo·car·y·no·sis

poi·ki·lo·cyte
    teardrop p.

poi·ki·lo·cy·the·mia

poi·ki·lo·cy·to·sis

poi·ki·lo·der·ma·tous

poi·ki·lo·der·mic

poi·ki·lo·throm·bo·cyte

point
    biologic end marker p's

pol gene

pol·ox·a·mer
    p. 188

poly

poly·ad·e·no·ma

poly·ad·e·no·ma·to·sis

poly·chro·ma·sia

poly·chro·ma·tia

poly·chro·ma·to·cy·to·sis

poly·chro·ma·to·phil·ia

poly·chro·ma·to·phil·ic

poly·chro·ma·to·sis

poly·chro·me·mia

poly·chro·mo·phil·ia

poly·clo·nal

poly·cyte

poly·cy·the·mia
    absolute p.
    appropriate p.
    benign p.
    compensatory p.
    p. hypertonica
    inappropriate p.
    myelopathic p.
    primary p.
    relative p.
    p. rubra
    p. rubra vera
    secondary p.
    splenomegalic p.
    spurious p.
    stress p.
    p. vera

poly·em·bry·o·ma

poly·em·bry·o·ny

poly·en·do·crine

poly·en·do·cri·no·ma

poly·es·tra·di·ol phos·phate

poly·eth·y·lene gly·col

poly-L-ly·sine

poly·morph

poly·mor·phism
    DNA p.
    genetic p.
    Malmö p.
    Pvu II p.

poly·mor·pho·nu·cle·ar
    filament p.
    nonfilament p.

poly·my·al·gia
    p. rheumatica

poly·myo·si·tis
    paraneoplastic p.

poly·nu·cle·ar

poly·o·ma

pol·yp
    adenomatous p.
    colonic p.
    colorectal p.
    Cronkhite-Canada p.
    diminutive p.
    duodenal p.
    epithelial p.
    familial adenomatous p's
    fundic gland p.
    gastric p.
    gastrointestinal p.
    gelatinous p.
    hamartomatous p.
    hyperplastic p.
    index p.
    inflammatory p.
    inflammatory fibroid p.
    juvenile p's
    malignant p.
    nasal p.
    neoplastic p.
    pedunculated p.
    Peutz-Jeghers p.
    retention p's
    sessile p.
    villous adenomatous p's

poly·pec·to·my
    colonoscopic p.

poly·pep·tide
    endothelial cell macro-
      phage activating p.
      (EMAP)
    vasoactive intestinal p.
      (VIP)

poly·pep·ti·de·mia

poly·phy·let·ic

poly·phy·le·tism

poly·phy·le·tist

poly·poi·do·sis

poly·po·sis
    adenomatous p.
    adenomatous p. coli
    familial p.
    familial adenomatous p.
    familial p. coli
    hamartomatous p.
    juvenile p.
    multiple colonic p.

poly·va·lent
    p. chloride

poly·vi·nyl·chlo·ride

POMP
    6-mercaptopurine, vincris-
      tine, methotrexate, and
      prednisone

pon·ceau S

pool

pop·u·la·tion
    cell p.

por·fi·ro·my·cin

po·ro·ma

por·phy·ria
    erythropoietic p.

por·phy·rin·emia

por·phy·ryl

port
    Groshong p.
    Hickman subcutaneous p.
    IMPLANTOFIX p.
    infusion p.
    subcutaneous p.

Port-A-Cath

Por·ta·lac

por·tog·ra·phy
    arterial p.
    CT arterial p.

post·al·bu·min

post·mas·tec·to·my

post·ra·di·a·tion

post·re·mis·sion

pot·as·se·mia

po·tas·si·um
   p. acetate
   p. bicarbonate
   p. chloride
   p. citrate
   p. dichromate
   p. ferrocyanide
   p. gluconate
   p. gluconate, p. citrate,
     and ammonium chloride
   p. and sodium phosphates

po·ten·tial
   zeta p.

po·ten·ti·a·tion

pouch
   gastric reservoir p.

pow·der
   talcum p.

pow·er
   carbon dioxide-combining
     p.
   CO_2-combining p.

PPACK
   D-phenylalanyl-L-prolyl-L-
     arginyl-chloromethyl ke-
     tone

PR
   partial remission
   partial response
   pathology report
   progesterone receptor

PRDI
   positive regulatory domain
     I

PRDII
   positive regulatory domain
     II

pre·ad·i·po·cyte

pre·can·cer

pre·can·cer·ous

pre·car·cin·o·gen

pre·car·ci·nom·a·tous

pre·cu·ne·us

pre·cur·sor
   amine p.
   granulopoietic p.
   leukocyte p.
   myeloid p.
   p. stem cell
   transglutaminase p.

PRED
   prednisone

Pred
   prednisone

Pred·a·ject-50

Pred·a·lone T.B.A.

Pre·date

Pred·cor

Pred·i·cort

pred·ni·mus·tine

pred·nis·o·lone

pred·ni·sone

preg·nan·cy
   molar p.

pre·in·va·sive

pre·kal·li·kre·in
   plasma p.

pre·leu·ke·mia

pre·leu·ke·mic

Pre·lone

pre·ma·lig·nant

Prem·a·rin

pre·mono·cyte

pre·my·elo·blast

pre·my·elo·cyte

prep·a·ra·tion
   Tzanck p.

pre·sen·ta·tion
   antigen p.

pre·ser·va·tion
   sphincter p.

pre-spleen

pre·throm·bin

pre·throm·bot·ic

Price
   P.-Jones curve
   P.-Jones method

Pril·o·sec

prim·a·quine

prim·a·quine phos·phate

primed

prim·ing

Prin·gle
   P's disease

Pro-50

pro·ac·cel·er·in

proACTH/LPH
   C3 p. (C3PA)

Pro·bal·an

probe
   biotinylated p.
   cDNA p.
   DNA p.
   DX13 p.
   St14 p.

pro·ben·e·cid

pro·bu·col

PROC
   procarbazine

Proc
   procarbazine

Proc AACR
   Proceedings of the Ameri-
   can Association for Can-
   cer Research

pro·car·ba·zine
   p. hydrochloride

pro·car·cin·o·gen

Proc ASCO
   Proceedings of the Ameri-
   can Society of Clinical
   Oncology

pro·ce·dure
   Billroth p.
   limb-sparing p.
   Shiu p.
   Whipple p.

Pro·ceed·ings of the Amer·i·
   can As·so·ci·a·tion for Can·
   cer Re·search

Pro·ceed·ings of the Amer·i·
   can So·ci·ety of Clin·i·cal
   On·col·o·gy

pro·chlor·per·a·zine

pro·co·ag·u·lant

pro·con·ver·tin

proc·to·co·lec·to·my
   total p.

proc·to·sig·moi·dec·to·my
   transanal abdominal
   transanal p.

proc·to·sig·moi·dos·co·py

proc·tot·o·my

Pro·cy·tox

Pro·De·po

Pro·di·em Plain

Pro·drox

prod·uct
   blood p's
   contact activation p.

prod·uct *(continued)*
    fibrin degradation p's
    fibrinolytic split p's
    fibrin split p.
    plasma p's
    plasma-derived p.

pro·duc·tion
    ectopic hormone p.

pro·eryth·ro·blast

pro·eryth·ro·cyte

pro·fi·bri·nol·y·sin
    antigenic p.

pro·fil·in

pro·gen·i·tor
    erythroid p.
    hematopoietic p.
    T-cell p.

pro·ges·te·rone

pro·ges·te·rone-re·cep·tor
  pos·i·tive

pro·ges·tin
    antitumor p.

pro·go·no·ma
    melanotic p.

pro·gram
    chemotherapy p.

pro·gran·u·lo·cyte

pro·gres·sion
    tumor p.

pro·kine

pro·lac·tin

pro·lac·ti·no·ma

pro·leu·ko·cyte

pro·lif·er·a·tion
    adventitial p.
    atypical vascular p.
    cell p.
    cellular p.
    endothelial p.

pro·lif·er·a·tion *(continued)*
    stromal p.
    vascular p.

pro·lif·er·a·tive

pro·line

Pro·loid

pro·lym·pho·cyte

pro·lym·pho·cyt·ic

pro·lym·pho·cy·toid

ProMACE
    prednisone, methotrexate, doxorubicin, cyclophosphamide, etoposide

ProMACE-CytaBOM
    prednisone, methotrexate, doxorubicin, cyclophosphamide, etoposide, cytarabine, bleomycin, vincristine, methotrexate

ProMACE-MOPP
    prednisone, methotrexate, doxorubicin, cyclophosphamide, etoposide, mechlorethamine, vincristine, procarbazine, prednisone

pro·mega·karyo·cyte

Pro·meth

pro·meth·a·zine

pro·mis·cu·i·ty
    lineage p.

pro·mi·to·sis

pro·mono·cyte

prom·on·to·ry

pro·mo·ter
    genetic p.

pro·mo·tion

pro·my·elo·cyte

pro·my·elo·cyt·ic

pro·nor·mo·blast

pro·pep·tide
   prothrombin p.

pro·per·din

pro·plas·ma·cyte

prop·y·lene
   p. oxide

Pro·ra·zin

Pro·rex

pro·ru·bri·cyte

pros·ta·cy·clin

pros·ta·glan·din

pros·ta·glan·din G/H syn·thase

pros·tate

pros·ta·tec·to·my
   radical p.
   retropubic radical p.

pros·ta·to·cys·tec·to·my

Pros·tin E2

pro·te·ase
   calcium-activated neutral p.

pro·tein
   p. A
   acute phase p's
   bcr-abl fusion p.
   Bence Jones p.
   p. C
   p. Ca
   carrier p.
   C4 binding p.
   CCAAT displacement p.
   Charcot-Leyden crystal p.
   contractile p.
   C-reactive p.
   G p.
   gag-abl fusion p.

pro·tein *(continued)*
   gag-fps fusion p.
   glial fibrillary acidic p.
   Glu-4 p.
   granule membrane p. (GMP-140)
   granulocyte chemotactic p. (GCP)
   p. Gs
   heat shock p. (Hsp)
   human p. S
   latent membrane p. (LMP)
   leech antiplatelet p.
   M p.
   macrophage inflammatory p. (MIP)
   macrophage inflammatory p. 1
   macrophage inflammatory p. 2
   myeloma p.
   nuclear p.
   octomer binding p.
   placental anticoagulant p. (PAP)
   plasma p's
   platelet activation–dependent granule–external membrane p. (PADGEM)
   platelet basic p.
   rattlesnake venom p.
   p. S
   S p.
   S-100 p.
   serum p's
   vitamin K–dependent p.

pro·tein·ase
   serine p.

pro·tein·emia
   Bence Jones p.

pro·tein ki·nase

pro·tein ki·nase A

pro·tein ki·nase C

pro·tein·uria
   Bence Jones p.

pro·te·ol·y·sis

Pro·tha·zine

pro·throm·bin
    p. *Barcelona*
    p. *Brussels*
    p. *Cardeza*
    p. *Houston*
    p. *Madrid*
    p. *Metz*
    p. *Molise*
    p. *Quick*
    p. *San Juan I*
    p. *San Juan II*

pro·throm·bin·ase
    extrinsic p.
    intrinsic p.

pro·throm·bi·no·gen·ic

pro·throm·bi·no·pe·nia

pro·thy·mo·cyte

pro·to·col
    Group C (Treatment IND)
      p.
    M-2 p.
    T-10 p.
    T-12 p.
    treatment p.

pro·to·heme

pro·to·he·min

pro·to-on·co·gene
    c-*fms* p.
    c-*fos* p.
    c-*raf* p.
    c-*ras* p.

Pro·to·pam

pro·to·plasm

pro·to·plas·mic

pro·to·por·phyr·ia

Pro·vera

PRO·VID·ER PLUS pump

pro·vi·rus

Prow·er
    P. factor

Prus·sian blue re·ac·tion

PS
    pathological stage

psam·mo·car·ci·no·ma

psam·mo·ma

psam·mo·sar·co·ma

PSCT
    peripheral stem cell trans-
      plantation

pseu·do·ag·glu·ti·na·tion

pseu·do·bac·il·lus

pseu·do·car·ci·no·ma

pseu·do·car·ci·nom·a·tous

pseu·do·eo·sin·o·phil
    chemotherapy-induced p.

pseu·do·hem·ag·glu·ti·na·
    tion

pseu·do·he·mo·phil·ia

pseu·do·hy·po·na·tre·mia

pseu·do–Ka·po·si sarcoma

pseu·do·leu·ke·mia

pseu·do·lym·pho·ma
    ocular p.

pseu·do·ma·lig·nan·cy

pseu·do·mel·a·no·ma

pseu·do·met·he·mo·glo·bin

Pseu·do·mo·nas

pseu·do·mu·ci·nous

pseu·do·neo·plasm

pseu·do-ovum

pseu·do·pal·i·sade

pseu·do·poly·cy·the·mia

pseu·do·re·sponse

pseu·do·ro·sette

pseu·do·sar·co·ma

pseu·do·sar·com·a·tous

pseu·do·struc·ture

pseu·do·throm·bo·cy·to·pe·nia

pseu·do·tu·mor
  inflammatory p.

pseu·do·vac·u·ole

pseu·do–von Wil·le·brand disease

psi·co·fur·a·nine

pso·ri·a·sis

PSTT
  placental site trophoblastic tumor

PSU
  primary site undetermined

psyl·li·um
  p. hydrophilic mucilloid

PTA
  plasma thromboplastin antecedent (blood coagulation Factor XI)

PTBD
  percutaneous transhepatic biliary drainage

PTC
  plasma thromboplastin component (blood coagulation Factor IX)

PTD
  photodynamic therapy

PTH
  parathyroid hormone

P53 tu·mor sup·pres·sor gene

Pud·lak
  Hermansky-P. syndrome

Pul·mo·lite

pump
  Abbott-Parker LifeCare 1500 p.
  ambulatory infusion p.
  Autosyringe p.
  balloon p.
  chemoinfusion p.
  Cormed p.
  Cormed II p.
  Cormed III p.
  Deltec-Pharmacia CADD p.
  external chemotherapy p.
  Graseby p.
  implantable chemoinfusion p.
  implanted infusion p.
  Infumed p.
  Infumed 200 p.
  Infusaid p.
  infusion p.
  Infusor p.
  Medtronic p.
  microvolume infusion p.
  nonvolumetric p.
  Pancretec 2000 p.
  peristaltic p.
  portable infusion p.
  PROVIDER PLUS p.
  syringe-cassette p.
  totally implantable chemoinfusion p.
  totally implantable chemotherapy p.
  Travenol Infusor p.
  volumetric p.

purged

purg·ing
  bone marrow p.

pu·rin·emia

pu·rin·emic

pu·rine-nu·cleo·side phos·
   phor·y·lase

pu·rine-nu·cleo·side phos·
   phor·y·lase de·fi·cien·cy

Pu·rine·thol

pu·ro·my·cin

pur·pu·ra
   allergic p.
   anaphylactoid p.
   chemical-induced p.
   cushingoid p.
   p. fulminans
   hypergammaglobulinemic
      p.
   hyperglobulinemic p. of
      Waldenström
   idiopathic thrombocyto-
      penic p.
   post-transfusion p.
   thrombotic thrombocyto-
      penic p.
   touch p.

PUVA
   psoralen-ultraviolet A

PVB
   cisplatin, vinblastine, and
      bleomycin

Pvu II poly·mor·phism

py·elog·ra·phy

pyk·no·cyte

pyk·no·cy·to·ma

pyk·no·cy·to·sis

pyo·my·o·ma

pyo·sap·re·mia

pyo·tox·in·emia

py·ra·zo·fur·in

Pyr·i·ben·za·mine

pyr·i·dox·ine
   p. hydrochloride

py·rim·i·dine
   p. dimer

py·ro·gen
   endogenous p.
   exogenous p's
   leukocytic p.

py·ro·glob·u·lin·emia

py·rol·y·sis

py·ro·nin
   p. B

py·ro·poi·ki·lo·cy·to·sis
   hereditary p.

py·ru·vate ki·nase (PK)

py·ru·vate ki·nase (PK) de·fi·
   cien·cy, eryth·ro·cyte

py·ru·ve·mia

py·ryl·amine

Q-Port

quad·ran·tec·to·my

Ques·tran

Quey·rat
    erythroplasia of Q.

Quick
    Q's test

Qui·ess

quin·a·crine hy·dro·chlo·ride

Quin·ton catheter

r
   recombinant

RA
   refractory anemia

Raaf
   R. catheter

ra·di·a·tion
   cobalt r.
   ionizing r.
   photon r.
   ultraviolet r.

Ra·di·a·tion Ther·a·py On·col·o·gy Group

ra·dio·bi·ol·o·gy

ra·dio·car·ci·no·gen·e·sis

ra·dio·con·ju·gate

ra·dio·cur·a·bil·i·ty

ra·dio·der·ma·ti·tis

ra·dio·epi·der·mi·tis

ra·dio·epi·the·li·tis

ra·dio·gold

ra·dio·graph
   chest r.

ra·di·og·ra·phy
   plain chest r.

ra·dio·im·mu·no·as·say

ra·dio·im·mu·no·con·ju·gate

ra·dio·im·mu·no·dif·fu·sion

ra·dio·im·mu·no·elec·tro·pho·re·sis

ra·dio·im·mu·no·lo·cal·iza·tion

ra·dio·im·mu·no·pre·cip·i·ta·tion

ra·dio·im·mu·no·sor·bent

ra·dio·io·dine

ra·dio·iso·tope

ra·dio·la·bel·ing

ra·di·ol·o·gy
   interventional r.

ra·dio·lu·mi·nes·cence
   single photon r.

ra·dio·nu·clide

ra·dio·phos·pho·rus

ra·dio·pro·tec·tion

ra·dio·pro·tec·tor

ra·dio·re·sis·tance

ra·dio·re·sis·tant

ra·dio·re·spon·sive

ra·dio·re·spon·sive·ness

ra·dio·sen·si·tive

ra·dio·sen·si·tiv·i·ty

ra·dio·sen·si·ti·zer
   hypoxic cell r.

ra·dio·sur·gery
   stereotactic r.

ra·dio·ther·a·py
   continuous, hyperfraction-
      ated, accelerated r.
      (CHART)
   external beam r.
   fractionated r.
   involved-field r.
   partial-brain r.
   single-dose r.
   split-course r.
   whole abdominal r.
   whole-brain r.

Ra·dio·ther·a·py On·col·o·
gy Group

ra·don
r. daughters

RAEB
refractory anemia with ex-
cess of blasts

RAEBIT
refractory anemia with ex-
cess of blasts in transformation

RAH
regressing atypical histio-
cytosis

Rai stag·ing (for chronic
lymphocytic leukemia)

Rai·nier
hemoglobin R.

ra·ni·ti·dine

Rap·pa·port
R. classification (for non-
Hodgkin's lymphoma)

RARS
refractory anemia with
ringed sideroblasts

rate
erythrocyte sedimentation
r. (ESR)
five-year survival r.
Westergren sedimentation
r.

Rath·ke
R's pouch
R's tumor

ra·tio
cell color r.
fasting insulin:glucose r.
zeta sedimentation r.
(ZSR)

Ray·naud
R's phenomenon

RC-1 (renal carcinoma) cell
line

rcf
ristocetin cofactor

RCS
reticulum cell sarcoma

re·ac·tion
acute phase r.
allograft r.
anaphylactic r.
antigen-antibody r.
antiglobulin r.
Bordet and Gengou r.
complement fixation r.
conglutination r.
cross r.
cytochemical r.
erythrocyte sedimentation
r.
graft-vs.-host r.
Haber-Weiss r.
hemagglutination-inhibi-
tion r.
hemolytic r.
Hopkins-Cole r.
hypersensitivity r.
indophenol r.
leukemic r.
leukemoid r.
mixed leukocyte r.
mixed lymphocyte r.
mononuclear cell r.
Nadi r.
oxidase r.
peroxidase r.
platelet basic r.
platelet release r.
polymerase chain r.
Prussian blue r.
sedimentation r.
serological r.
serum r.
serum sickness–like r.
transfusion r.

re·ac·ti·va·tion
r. of serum

re·ac·tor
continuous flow r.

re·a·gent
ADP r.
collagen r.
Desferal-bound iron r.
Drabkin's r.
epinephrine r.
iron color r.
lactate r.
peroxidase indicator r.
platelet aggregation r.
red cell lysing r.
ristocetin r.
Schiff's r.
UIBC r.

re·ar·range·ment
gene r.

re·bound
heparin r.

re·can·al·iza·tion

re·cep·tor
adrenergic r's
androgen r.
B cell antigen r's
C3b r
complement r's
cytoadhesin r.
effector cell protease r.-1
(EPR-1)
eicosanoid r.
epidermal growth factor r.
estrogen r.
Fc r's
gamma-delta T cell r.
glucocorticoid r.
growth factor r.
homing r.
5-HT (serotonin) r.
IgE r's
laminin r.
lymphocyte homing r.
(LHR)
progesterone r.
RGD recognition r's

re·cep·tor *(continued)*
serotonin r.
T cell antigen r's
transferrin r.
tumor necrosis factor r.
(TNFR)

re·cep·tor-neg·a·tive

re·cip·i·ent
universal r.

re·cog·nin

re·com·bin·ase

re·cov·ery
platelet r.

re·cur·rence
anastomotic r.
local r.
tumor r.

re·cur·rent

red
neutral r.
r. O
toluene r.

re·duc·er
Fiske & SubbaRow r.

Reed
R. cells
R.-Hodgkin disease
R.-Sternberg cells
Sternberg-R. cells

Rees
R. and Ecker diluting fluid
R.-Ecker solution

re·flec·tion
peritoneal r.

re·frac·tor·i·ness
platelet r.

Re·gan
R. isoenzyme

Re·gaud
R. pattern

reg·i·men
    antiemetic r.
    Bonn r.
    chemotherapy r.
    conditioning r.
    conventional-dose r.
    Cooper r.
    high-dose r.
    Indiana University r.
    low-dose r.
    Malmö r.
    modified MSKCC r.
    MSKCC r.
    standard-dose r.
    Wayne State r.

re·gion
    breakpoint cluster r. (bcr)
    C_H r.
    C_L r.
    constant (C) r.
    hinge r.
    homology r's
    hypervariable r's
    locus activation r.
    locus control r.
    major breakpoint r. (mbr)
    minor cluster r. (mcr)
    promoter r.
    variable (V) r.
    V_H r.
    V_L r.

re·gres·sion
    tumor r.

reg·u·la·tion
    gene r.

re·ha·bil·i·ta·tion
    cosmetic r.

Reid
    R. factor

Reil·ly
    Alder-R. anomaly
    R's granulations

re·jec·tion
    graft r.

re·jec·tion *(continued)*
    transplant r.

re·lapse
    bone marrow r.
    central nervous system r.
    hematologic r.
    testicular r.

re·mis·sion
    clinical r.
    clonal r.
    complete r.
    cytogenetic r.
    r. induction
    partial r.
    pathologic r.
    spontaneous r.

re·peat
    long terminal r.

re·place·ment
    blood component r.
    platelet r.
    red blood cell r.

re·pop·u·la·tion

Rep-Pred

rep·til·ase

RES
    reticuloendothelial system

res·cue
    citrovorum r.
    leucovorin r.

re·sect

re·sec·ta·ble

re·sec·tion
    abdominoperineal r.
    coloanal r.
    palliative r.
    pulmonary r.
    rim r.
    sigmoid r.

re·serve
    alkali r.

re·serve *(continued)*
    alkaline r.
    bone marrow r.

re·ser·voir
    Ommaya r.

re·sid·u·al

res·in
    podophyllum r.

re·sis·tance
    cross-r.
    cytokinetic drug r.
    drug r.
    heparin r.
    multidrug r.
    pleiotropic r.
    pleiotropic drug r.

re·sorp·tion
    bone r.

re·spond·er

re·sponse
    antibody r.
    cellular r.
    complete r.
    early r.
    host r.
    immune r.
    inflammatory r.
    partial r.
    reticulocyte r.
    tissue r.
    tumor r.

rest
    aberrant r.

re·stag·ing

re·stric·tion

re·te·the·li·o·ma

re·tic·u·lo·cyte

re·tic·u·lo·cy·to·gen·ic

re·tic·u·lo·cy·to·pe·nia

re·tic·u·lo·cy·to·sis

re·tic·u·lo·en·do·the·li·o·ma

re·tic·u·lo·en·do·the·li·o·sis
    leukemic r.

re·tic·u·lo·his·ti·o·cy·to·ma

re·tic·u·lo·his·ti·o·cy·to·sis

re·tic·u·lo·ma

re·tic·u·lo·pe·nia

re·tic·u·lo·sis
    familial hemophagocytic r.
    familial histiocytic r.
    histiocytic medullary r.
    midline malignant r.
    polymorphic r.

Rol·let
    R's stroma

ret·i·no·blas·to·ma
    familial r.

ret·i·noid

re·trac·tion
    clot r.

ret·ro·vi·rus

rev gene

rex gene

RFS
    relapse-free survival

rG-CSF
    granulocyte colony stimu-
       lating factor, recombi-
       nant

rGM-CSF
    granulocyte macrophage-
       colony stimulating factor,
       recombinant E

Rh_{null}

rhab·doid

rhab·do·myo·blas·to·ma

rhab·do·myo·chon·dro·ma

rhab·do·my·o·ma

rhab·do·myo·myx·o·ma

rhab·do·myo·sar·co·ma
    alveolar r.
    embryonal r.
    ocular r.
    parameningeal r.
    truncal r.

rhab·do·sar·co·ma

Rheu·ma·trex

Rh fac·tor

rhi·zot·o·my
    cranial nerve r.

Rh-null syn·drome

Rho·do·pseu·do·mo·nas
    R. sphaeroides

RHR
    resectable, high-risk

Rib·bert
    R's theory

ri·bo·fla·vin

ri·bo·prine

RIC
    radioimmunoconjugate

Rich·ter
    Clough and R's syndrome
    R's syndrome

ri·cin
    anti-MY9–blocked r.
    B₄-blocked r.

RID
    radial immunodiffusion

Rie·del
    R's anomaly

Rie·der
    R. cell leukemia
    R's lymphocyte

RIF
    rosette-inhibiting factor

rIFN
    interferon recombinant

rIL
    interleukin recombinant

ring
    Waldeyer's r.

Ring·ertz
    R. classification (for astro-
    cytomas)
    R.-Burger classification
    (for astrocytomas)

RIPA
    ristocetin-induced platelet
    agglutination
    ristocetin-induced platelet
    aggregation

ris·to·ce·tin

RMS (Ruvalcaba-Myrhe-
    Smith) syn·drome

RNA (ribonucleic acid)
    antisense RNA

Ro·ba·late

Roche
    R.-Wainer-Thissen meth-
    odology

Rof·er·on-A

Romme·laere
    R's sign

Ro·sen·thal
    R. fiber
    R. syndrome

ro·sette
    E r.
    EAC r.
    Homer Wright r.

Roth·mund
    R.-Thomson syndrome

Ro·tor
    R. syndrome

Rot·ter
    R's nodes

rou·leau *pl.* rou·leaux

Rown·tree
    Levy, R., and Marriott's
        method

Roy·chlor

Roy·o·nate

RT
    radiation therapy
    radiotherapy

RT + 5-Fu
    radiation therapy and 5-
        fluorouracil

RTOG
    Radiation Therapy Oncol-
        ogy Group

Ru·bex

ru·bid·a·zone

ru·bid·o·my·cin

ru·bri·blast

ru·bri·cyte

rule
    Lossen's r.

Rum-K

Run·dles
    R.-Falls syndrome

Rus·sell
    R. bodies
    R's viper venom

Ru·val·ca·ba
    R.-Myrhe-Smith syndrome

Rye clas·si·fi·ca·tion (for
    Hodgkin's disease)

Sa·bin
    megaloblast of S.

Sah·li
    S's method

St. Ann-Mayo clas·si·fi·ca·tion (for astrocytomas)

St. Jude Chil·dren's Re·search

SAKK
    Swiss Group for Clinical
    Cancer Research

sal·i·cyl·emia

Sal·mon
    Durie-S. staging (for mye-
    loma)

Sal·mo·nel·la
    S. minnesota

Sal·o·mon
    S's test

sal·pin·go-ooph·o·rec·to·my

sal·vage
    limb s.

San·der·son
    Murchison-S. syndrome

San·do·sta·tin

San·ford
    S's test

san·gui·fa·cient

san·gui·fi·ca·tion

san·guine

san·guin·e·ous

san·gui·no·poi·et·ic

san·gui·nous

sar·co·car·ci·no·ma

sar·co·en·chon·dro·ma

sar·coid
    Spiegler-Fendt s.

L-sar·co·ly·sin

sar·co·ma *pl.* sar·co·mas, sar·co·ma·ta
    Abernethy's s.
    adipose s.
    AIDS-associated Kaposi's
    s.
    alveolar soft part s.
    ameloblastic s.
    B cell immunoblastic s.
    benign soft tissue s.
    bone s.
    botryoid s.
    s. botryoides
    bronchogenic s.
    chloromatous s.
    chondroblastic s.
    chondroblastic osteogenic
    s.
    clear cell s.
    s. colli uteri hydropicum
    papillare
    colorectal s.
    deciduocellular s.
    embryonal s.
    endometrial s.
    endometrial stromal s.
    epithelioid s.
    esophageal s.
    Ewing's s.
    extraosseous Ewing's s.
    fallopian tube s.
    fascial s.
    fibroblastic s.
    fibroblastic osteogenic s.
    giant cell s.
    granulocytic s.
    head and neck s.
    Hodgkin's s.
    idiopathic multiple pig-
    mented hemorrhagic s.

sar·co·ma *(continued)*
   immunoblastic s. of B cells
   immunoblastic s. of T cells
   Kaposi's s.
   Kupffer cell s.
   leukocytic s.
   lymphatic s.
   melanotic s.
   mixed cell s.
   multifocal sclerosing os-
      teogenic s.
   multiple idiopathic hemor-
      rhagic s.
   osteoblastic s.
   osteogenic s.
   osteoid s.
   osteolytic s.
   ovarian s.
   parosteal s.
   polymorphous s.
   postirradiation s.
   postirradiation osteogenic
      s.
   pseudo–Kaposi s.
   retroperitoneal s.
   serocystic s.
   small cell osteogenic s.
   small round cell s.
   soft tissue s.
   spindle-cell s.
   stromal s.
   synovial s.
   synovial cell s.
   telangiectatic s.
   telangiectatic osteogenic s.
   undifferentiated s.
   uterine s.
   vaginal s.
   vascular s.
   vulvar s.

sar·co·ma·gen·ic

sar·co·ma·ta

sar·co·ma·toid

sar·co·ma·to·sis
   s. cutis
   general s.

sar·co·ma·tous

sar·gra·mos·tim

sat·el·li·tism
   platelet s.

sat·el·li·to·sis
   perineuronal s.

sat·u·ra·tion
   oxygen s.

sau·cer·iza·tion

SC
   secretory component

SCAB
   streptozocin, lomustine,
      doxorubicin, and bleomy-
      cin

scale
   American Joint Commit-
      tee on Cancer Perform-
      ance Status S.
   CALGB (Cancer and Leu-
      kemia Group B) toxicity
      s.

scan
   baseline s.
   bone s.
   coronal s.
   gallium radionuclide s.
   sagittal s.

Scan·di·na·vi·an My·co·sis
   Fun·goid·es Study Group

Scan·di·na·vi·an My·co·sis
   Fun·goid·es Study Group
   stag·ing

scan·ning
   bone s.
   delayed iodine s.
   gallium s.
   radionuclide s.
   technetium s.
   thallium s.

SCBE
    single-contrast barium
      enema

SCC
    squamous cell cancer

SCCHN
    squamous cell carcinoma
      of the head and neck

Schal·fi·jew
    S's test

Schenk
    Churukian-S. stain

Schiff
    periodic acid–S. stain
    S's reagent

Schil·ling
    S's leukemia

schis·to·cyte

schis·to·cy·to·sis

schizo·cyte

schizo·cy·to·sis

Schmin·cke
    S. pattern
    S. tumor

Schül·ler
    S's disease

Schultz
    S's angina
    S's disease
    S. syndrome
    Werner-S. disease

Schul·tze
    S's indophenol oxidase test

Schwach·man
    S. syndrome
    S.-Diamond syndrome

Schwann
    S.-cell tumor

schwan·no·gli·o·ma

schwan·no·ma
    granular cell s.

Schwartz
    Watson-S. test

SCID
    severe combined immuno-
      deficiency

scin·tig·ra·phy
    bone s.

scir·rhoid

scir·rho·ma
    s. caminianorum

scir·rhous

scir·rhus

SCLC
    small cell lung cancer

scle·ro·sar·co·ma

scle·ro·sis
    nodular s.

scle·ro·ther·a·py

Scott
    S. syndrome

screen
    tangent s.

screen·ing
    donor s.

SCT
    stem cell transplantation

scur·vy

SD
    stable disease

SD (serologically defined) an·
  ti·gens

Se·at·tle
    hemoglobin S.

se·cond-look

sed·i·men·ta·tion
    erythrocyte s.

seed·ing
    tumor s.

SEG
    Southeastern Cancer
        Study Group

seg·men·ta·tion
    nuclear s.

Sel·dane

se·lec·tion
    immunoabsorbtive s.

sem·i·no·ma
    anaplastic s.
    mediastinal s.
    ovarian s.
    spermatocytic s.
    spermocytic s.

se·mus·tine

Sen·e·gal haplotype

se·nes·cent

sen·si·ti·za·tion
    autoerythrocyte s.
    Rh s.

sen·si·tiz·er
    hypoxic s.
    hypoxic cell s.
    nonhypoxic cell s.

SEOG
    Southeastern Cancer
        Study Group
    Southeastern Oncology
        Group

sep·a·ra·tion
    immunomagnetic s.

sep·a·ra·tor
    cell s.

Seph·a·dex

sep·sis
    s. agranulocytica

se·quence
    Drickamer s.
    E-box s.
    enhancer s.
    gamma-(312–324) s.
    linear sebaceous nevus s.
    neurocutaneous melanosis
        s.

se·quenc·ing
    direct s.

se·ques·tra·tion

se·ra

se·ral·bu·min

se·ries
    basophil s.
    basophilic s.
    eosinophil s.
    eosinophilic s.
    erythrocyte s.
    erythrocytic s.
    granulocyte s.
    granulocytic s.
    leukocytic s.
    lymphocyte s.
    lymphocytic s.
    monocyte s.
    monocytic s.
    myelocytic s.
    myeloid s.
    neutrophil s.
    neutrophilic s.
    plasmacyte s.
    plasmacytic s.
    thrombocyte s.
    thrombocytic s.
    UGI (upper gastrointes-
        tinal) s.

ser·ine ki·nase

ser·ine pro·te·ase

se·ro·al·bu·min·ous

se·ro·con·ver·sion

se·ro·con·vert

se·ro·glob·u·lin

se·ro·log·ic

se·ro·log·i·cal

se·rol·o·gist

se·rol·o·gy
    diagnostic s.

se·rol·y·sin

se·ro·neg·a·tive

se·ro·neg·a·tiv·i·ty

se·ro·pos·i·tive

se·ro·pos·i·tiv·i·ty

se·ro·prog·no·sis

se·ro·re·ac·tion

se·rose

sero·to·nin

se·rous

ser·pin

Ser·ra·tia
    S. marcescens

Ser·to·li
    S.-Leydig cell tumor

se·rum *pl.* se·rums, se·ra
    active s.
    anticomplementary s.
    antilymphocyte s. (ALS)
    blood s.
    blood grouping s's
    inactivated s.

ses·sile

Sé·zary
    S. cell

SGD
    specific granule deficiency

Shee·han
    S. syndrome

shift
    chloride s.
    s. to the left
    regenerative blood s.
    s. to the right

Shi·ma·da
    S. classification (of prognostic factors in neuroblastoma)

Shiu
    S. procedure

shock
    anaphylactic s.
    hematogenic s.
    hemorrhagic s.
    hypovolemic s.
    LPS-induced s.
    oligemic s.
    septic s.

shunt
    peritoneovenous s.

Sia
    S. test

SIADH
    syndrome of inappropriate antidiuretic hormone secretion

si·a·log·ra·phy

si·alo·trans·fer·ase

sick·le·mia

sick·le·mic

sick·ling

sick·ness
    serum s.

sid·ero·blast
    ring s.
    ringed s.

sid·ero·cyte

sid·ero·phage

sid·ero·phil·in

sid·ero·phore

sid·er·o·sis

sid·er·ot·ic

sids
    shared idiotypes

SId 4656 stro·mal cell line

SIG fam·i·ly

sig·moid

sig·moido·scope
    flexible s.

sig·moid·os·co·py

sign
    Leser-Trélat s.
    Lhermitte's s.
    Mosler's s.
    Rommelaere's s.
    Sterles' s.
    Troisier's s.

sig·nal
    accessory s.
    Il-1 accessory s.
    IL-6 accessory s.

sig·nal·ing

Si·lain-Gel

sil·i·ca

Sim·aal Gel

Sim·aal 2 Gel

si·meth·i·cone
    s., alumina, calcium car-
        bonate, and magnesia
    alumina, magnesia, and s.

si·meth·i·cone *(continued)*
    s., alumina, magnesium
        carbonate, and magnesia
    calcium carbonate and s.
    calcium carbonate, magne-
        sia, and s.
    magaldrate and s.

Si·mon
    Norton-S. hypothesis

Si·mon·ton
    S. method

si·nus *pl.* si·nus, si·nus·es
    paranasal s's

Sip·ple
    S's syndrome

Sis·ter Jo·seph
    S.J.'s nodule

Sis·ter Mary Jo·seph
    S.M.J. node

site
    antigen-binding s.
    antigen-combining s.
    binding s's
    transcription start s. (TSS)

Si·we
    Letterer-S. disease

skim·ming
    plasma s.

SK-MEL-37 (melanoma) cell
    line

Slo-Ni·a·cin

Slo-Phyl·lin

Slo-Pot 600

Sly
    S's syndrome

smear
    Pap s.
    Papanicolaou s.
    peripheral blood s.

Smith
    Ruvalcaba-Myhre-S. syn-
        drome

smok·ing
    passive s.

so·di·um
    alumina, magnesium tri-
        silicate, and s. bicarbon-
        ate
    s. ascorbate
    aspirin, s. bicarbonate,
        and citric acid
    s. barbital
    s. benzoate and s. phenyl-
        acetate
    s. chromate Cr 51
    s. dichloroacetate
    s. iodide I 131
    magnesium carbonate and
        s. bicarbonate
    s. metabisulfite
    s. monomercaptoundecahy-
        dro-closo-dodeca-borate
    s. pertechnetate Tc 99m
    s. phosphate P 32
    s. polystyrene sulfonate
    potassium and s. phos-
        phates
    s. thiosulfate

Solu-Cor·tef

Solu-Med·rol

so·lu·tion
    acid hematoxylin s.
    acid molybdate s.
    alkaline buffer s.
    barium hydroxide s.
    buffer s.
    DHEA standard s.
    Drabkin's s.
    fluorouracil topical s.
    Fonio's s.
    glucose standard s.
    glutaraldehyde s.
    Gowers' s.
    Hanks balanced salt s.

so·lu·tion *(continued)*
    Hayem's s.
    hematoxylin s., Gill No. 3
    lactate standard s.
    Mayer's hematoxylin s.
    p-nitrophenol standard s.
    pararosaniline s.
    phosphate-buffered saline
        s.
    phosphorus standard s.
    Rees-Ecker s.
    tartrate acid buffer s.
    tartrazine s.
    Toison's s.
    trypan blue s.
    Weigert's iron hematoxy-
        lin s.
    zinc sulfate s.

so·ma·to·stat·in

so·ma·to·stat·i·no·ma

so·no·gram

so·no·graph·ic

so·nog·ra·phy

sor·bi·tol-3-phos·phate

sort·er
    fluorescence-activated cell
        s. (FACS)

So·tos
    S. syndrome

Sou·lier
    Bernard-S. disease
    Bernard-S. syndrome

South·east·ern Can·cer Stu·
    dy Group

South·ern
    S. blot
    S. blot analysis

South·west·ern On·col·o·gy
    Group

Sout·tar
    S's tube

Span-Ni·a·cin

SPCA
    serum prothrombin con-
        version accelerator (blood
        coagulation factor VII)

SPECT
    single photon emission
        computed tomography

spec·trin
    α-s.

spec·tros·co·py
    magnetic resonance s.

sper·ma·to·cy·to·ma

sper·mo·cy·to·ma

sphe·ro·cyte

sphe·ro·cyt·ic

sphe·ro·cy·to·sis
    hereditary s.

sphe·ro·ma

sphin·go·lip·id

sphin·go·my·e·lin

Spie·gler
    S.-Fendt sarcoid

spi·rad·e·no·ma
    cylindromatous s.

spi·ro·ger·ma·ni·um

spi·ro·ma

spir·o·no·lac·tone
    s. and hydrochlorothiazide

spleen
    accessory s.
    hard-baked s.

sple·nec·to·my

splen·ic

sple·no·ma *pl.* sple·no·mas,
    sple·no·mata

sple·no·meg·a·ly
    hemolytic s.

sple·non·cus

SPN
    solid pulmonary nodule

spon·gio·blas·to·ma
    s. multiforme
    s. unipolare

spon·gio·cy·to·ma

spread
    lymphangitic s.
    tumor s.

S-100 pro·tein

SPS Sus·pen·sion

SSM
    superficial spreading mel-
        anoma

stage
    pathological s.

stag·ing
    AJCC/UICC s. (for colorec-
        tal cancer)
    Ann Arbor s. (for Hodg-
        kin's disease)
    Astler-Coller s. (for colo-
        rectal carcinoma)
    Binet s.
    Children's Cancer Study
        Group s. (for neuroblas-
        toma)
    Durie-Salmon s. (for mye-
        loma)
    Evans s. (for neuroblas-
        toma)
    FIGO s. (for ovarian can-
        cer)
    Indiana University s. (for
        testicular cancer)
    Jass s. (for rectal carci-
        noma)
    M.D. Anderson Hospital s.
        (for melanoma)
    Pediatric Oncology Group
        s. (for neuroblastoma)

stag·ing *(continued)*
    Rai s. (for chronic lympho-
      cytic leukemia)
    St. Jude Children's Re-
      search Hospital s. (for
      neuroblastoma)
    Scandinavian Mycosis
      Fungoides Study Group
      s.
    surgical s.
    TNM s.
    UICC (International
      Union Against Cancer) s.
    Whitmore s. (for prostate
      cancer)

stain
    acid phosphatase s.
    Churukian-Schenk s.
    cytochemical s.
    Fontana-Masson s.
    Giemsa s.
    Henner's s.
    iron s.
    Jenner's s.
    May-Grünwald s.
    mucicarmine s.
    naphthol AS-D acetate s.
    Papanicolaou's s.
    periodic acid–Schiff (PAS)
      s.
    peroxidase s.
    reticulocyte s.
    Sudan black s.
    tetrachrome s.
    Wright's s.
    Wright-Giemsa s.

stain·ing
    immunocytochemical s.
    impox (immunoperoxidase)
      s.

stan·o·zo·lol

starch
    hydroxyethyl s.

state
    immunodeficiency s.

state *(continued)*
    postspelenectomy s.
    prethrombotic s.
    thrombotic s.

sta·tus
    receptor s.

stau·ro·spor·ine

STC
    subtotal colectomy

ste·a·ral·de·hyde

ste·a·to·ma *pl.* ste·a·to·ma·
    ta, ste·a·to·mas

ste·a·to·ma·to·sis

Stein·brinck
    Chédiak-S.-Higashi anom-
      aly

Ste·met·ic

Ste·me·til

Ste·re·cyt

ster·e·ol·o·gy

ster·eo·tax·ic

Sterles
    S. sign

Stern·berg
    Reed-S. cells
    S's disease
    S's giant cells
    S.-Reed cells

ste·roid
    anabolic s.
    andrenogenic s.
    antitumor s.

Ste·wart
    S.-Treves syndrome

St^a gly·co·phor·in

Stil·phos·trol

Stim·ate

stim·u·la·tion
  antigenic s.
  dorsal column s.
  LPS s.

stim·u·lus *pl.* stim·u·li
  oncogenic s.

STLI
  subtotal lymphoid irradia-
    tion

sto·ma·to·cy·to·sis

sto·ma·to·tox·ic·i·ty
  direct s.
  indirect s.

stor·age
  blood s.
  blood component s.

strep·to·ni·grin

strep·to·zo·cin

strep·to·zo·to·cin

stress
  granulopoietic s.
  oxidating s.

stro·ma *pl.* stro·ma·ta
  fibrovascular s.
  pseudosarcomatous s.
  Rollet's s.

stro·mal

stro·mat·ic

stro·ma·tin

stro·ma·tol·y·sis

struc·ture
  kringle s.

stru·ma
  s. lipomatodes aberrata
    renis
  s. maligna
  s. nodosa

STU

Stu·art
  S. factor

study
  baseline s.
  cytogenetic s.
  immunoperoxidase s.
  Multi-institutional Osteo-
    sarcoma S.
  x-ray s.

stump
  cervical s.

Styp·ven
  S. time test

STZ
  streptozocin

Stz
  streptozocin

sub·ep·en·dy·mo·ma

sub·leu·ke·mic

sub·lym·phe·mia

sub·stag·ing

sub·stance
  α-s., alpha s.
  blood group s's
  H s.
  metachromatic s.
  no-threshold s's
  s. P
  reticular s.
  threshold s's
  thromboplastic s.
  thyrotropic s.
  zymoplastic s.

sub·stan·tia *pl.* sub·stan·tiae
  s. reticulofilamentosa

sub·sti·tu·tion
  C→T s.

su·cros·emia

su·dano·phil

su·dano·phil·ic

sug·ar
    blood s.

sul·cus *pl.* sul·ci
    superior pulmonary s.

sul·fate
    dermatan s.
    ferrous s.

sul·fat·emia

sulf·he·mo·glo·bin

sulf·he·mo·glo·bin·emia

sul·fin·py·ra·zone

sulf·met·he·mo·glo·bin

sul·fon·am·i·de·mia

sul·fur
    s. mustard

sul·in·dac

su·per·ox·ide

su·per·ox·ide dis·mu·tase
    s.d. (recombinant human)

su·per·ve·nos·i·ty

SUP-M2 (large cell lymphoma)
    cell line

sup·port
    nutritional s.

sup·pres·sion
    bone marrow s.

su·pra·glot·tis

su·pra·ten·to·ri·al

Su·pre·fact

sur·gery
    breast-conserving s.
    cytoreductive s.
    limb-sparing s.
    Mohs' s.
    palliative s.
    second-look s.

sur·veil·lance
    immune s.
    immunological s.

sur·vi·val
    disease-free s.
    median s.
    overall s.
    progression-free s.
    relapse-free s.

sus·pen·sion
    testolactone s., sterile

SVC
    superior vena cava

Sweet
    S's syndrome

Swiss Group for Clin·i·cal
    Can·cer Re·search

Swiss type agam·ma·glob·u·
    lin·emia

switch
    class s.

switch·ing
    hemoglobin s.

SWOG
    Southwest Oncology Group
    Southwestern Oncology
        Group

Syd·ney
    amended S. classification
    S. classification (for extra-
        ocular melanoma)
    S. line

Sym·mers
    Brill-S. disease
    S. disease

sym·path·i·co·blas·to·ma

sym·path·i·co·go·ni·o·ma

sym·pa·tho·blas·to·ma

sym·pa·tho·go·ni·o·ma

symp·tom
 esophagosalivary s.

syn·ap·to·phy·sin

syn·chro·ni·za·tion
 chemotherapeutic s.

syn·clit·ic

syn·clit·i·cism

syn·clit·ism
 s. malignum

syn·des·mo·ma
 −7 s.

syn·drome (see also under
 disease)
 Aase s.
 acquired immunodefi-
  ciency s. (AIDS)
 acute splenic sequestration
  s.
 Aldrich's s.
 anemia-neutropenia-lym-
  phocytosis s.
 anorexia-cachexia s.
 argentaffinoma s.
 ataxia-telangiectasia s.
 atypical myeloproliferative
  s.
 bare lymphocyte s.
 Bartter's s.
 Beckwith-Wiedemann s.
 Bernard-Soulier s. (BSS)
 big spleen s.
 Blackfan-Diamond s.
 Bloom s.
 bone marrow failure s's
 breast-ovarian cancer s.
 Buckley's s.
 cancer family s.
 carcinoid s.
 Chédiak-Higashi s.
 chronic lymphadenopathy
  s.
 Clough and Richter's s.
 cold agglutinin s.

syn·drome *(continued)*
 combined immunodefi-
  ciency s.
 Conn's s.
 Cowden's s.
 Cronkhite-Canada s.
 CRST s.
 Cushing's s.
 Cushing's s. medicamento-
  sus
 defibrination s.
 Degos' s.
 De Sanctis-Cacchione s.
 Diamond-Blackfan s.
 DiGeorge s.
 Di Guglielmo s.
 disuse s.
 Down s.
 Dresbach's s.
 Duncan's s.
 dyskeratosis congenita s.
 dysmyelopoietic s.
 dysplastic nevus s.
 ectopic ACTH s.
 Ehlers-Danlos s.
 eosinophilia-myalgia s.
 Evans's s.
 Faber's s.
 Fabry s.
 familial colon cancer s.
 Fanconi's s.
 Fanconi's pancytopenia s.
 Felty's s.
 feminizing s.
 flat adenoma s.
 focal cerebral s.
 focal intratentorial s.
 Gaisböck's s.
 Gardner's s.
 Gasser's s.
 giant platelet s.
 glioma-polyposis s.
 glucagonoma s.
 Good's s.
 Goodpasture's s.
 Gorlin's s.
 gray platelet s.
 Griscelli s.

syn·drome *(continued)*
Hare's s.
Hayem-Widal s.
hemolytic-uremic s.
hereditary nonpolyposis
  colorectal cancer s.
Hermansky-Pudlak s.
Hutchison s.
hypereosinophilic s.
hyperimmunoglobulinemia
  E s.
hyperviscosity s.
idiopathic flushing s.
Imerslund s.
Imerslund-Graesbeck s.
immunodeficiency s.
infratentorial s.
inhibitory s.
intravascular coagulation-
  fibrinolysis s.
Job s.
Josephs-Diamond-Blackfan
  s.
Kaznel's s. I
Kenny s.
Kostmann's s.
Langer-Giedion s.
lazy leukocyte s.
leukoerythroblastic s.
Li-Fraumeni s.
Louis-Bar s.
lymphocytosis-anemia-
  neutropenia s.
lymphoproliferative s.
Lynch s. (I and II)
Maffucci's s.
Malin's s.
Marchiafava-Micheli s.
Maroteaux-Lamy s.
masculinizing s.
Meigs' s.
Miller Fisher s.
Minkowski-Chauffard s.
Minot-von Willebrand s.
mononucleosis s.
Mosse's s.
mucosal neuroma s.
Muir s.

syn·drome *(continued)*
multiple exostoses s.
multiple hamartoma s.
multiple neuroma s.
MUO (metastasis of un-
  known origin) s.
Murchison-Sanderson s.
myasthenic s.
myelodysplastic s.
myelofibrosis-osteosclerosis
  s.
myeloproliferative s.
neurofibromatosis s.
nevoid basal cell carci-
  noma s.
nevoid basalioma s.
Nezelof s.
Oldfield's s.
osteochondromatosis s.
Pancoast's s.
pancytopenia-dysmelia s.
paraneoplastic s.
Paterson-Kelly s.
Peutz-Jeghers s.
Plummer-Vinson s.
preleukemic s.
pseudo-Felty's s.
13q s.
radial aplasia–thrombocy-
  topenia s.
Rh-null s.
Richter's s.
Roberts-SC phocomelia s.
Rosenthal s.
Rothmund-Thomson s.
Rotor's s.
Rundles-Falls s.
runting s.
Ruvalcaba-Myrhe-Smith s.
SBLA s.
Schultz s.
Schwachman s.
Schwachman-Diamond s.
Scott s.
s. of sea-blue histiocyte
serum sickness-like s.
Sézary s.
Sheehan's s.

syn·drome *(continued)*
  shoulder-hand s.
  Sipple's s.
  Sly s.
  Sotos' s.
  Stewart-Treves s.
  superior sulcus tumor s.
  superior vena cava s.
  Sweer's s.
  TAR (thrombocytopenia–absent radius) s.
  thrombocytopenia–absent radius (TAR) s.
  Torres' s.
  trisomy 8 s.
  trisomy 13 s.
  trisomy 18 s.
  Trousseau's s.
  tuberous sclerosis s.
  tumor lysis s.
  Turcot s.
  von Hippel-Lindau s.
  Waring blender s.
  Wermer's s.
  Werner s.
  Willebrand's s.
  Wiskott-Aldrich s.
  xeroderma pigmentosa s.
  X-linked lymphoproliferative s.
  Zanca's s.
  Zollinger-Ellison s.

syn·er·gism
  clinical s.

syn·er·gy

syn·ge·ne·ic

syn·ge·ne·sio·plas·tic

syn·ge·ne·sio·trans·plan·ta·tion

syn·graft

sy·no·vi·a·lo·ma

sy·no·vi·o·ma
  benign s.
  malignant s.

sy·no·vio·sar·co·ma

syn·the·tase

Syn·throid

Syn·to·ci·non

sy·rin·go·ad·e·no·ma

sy·rin·go·car·ci·no·ma

sy·rin·go·cys·tad·e·no·ma
  s. papilliferum

sy·rin·go·cys·to·ma

sy·rin·go·ma

sys·tem
  American Mycosis Fungoides Cooperative Group s. (for staging of mycosis fungoides)
  APUD s.
  Bak a/Bak b alloantigen s.
  Binet staging s. (for chronic lymphocytic leukemia)
  blood group s.
  Breslow s. (for melanoma staging)
  BSD hyperthermia s.
  buffer s.
  cardiopulmonary s.
  cardiovascular s.
  central nervous s. (CNS)
  Clark s. (for staging of melanoma)
  coagulation s.
  complement s.
  demarcation membrane s.
  endothelial s.
  fibrinolytic s.
  hematopoietic s.
  humoral amplification s's
  immune s.
  International Staging S. (INNS) (for neuroblastoma)
  lymphoid s.
  lymphoreticular s.

sys·tem *(continued)*
    macrophage s.
    mononuclear phagocyte s.
     (MPS)
    natural killer s.
    ONCOCIN s.
    open canicular s.
    PDQ s.

sys·tem *(continued)*
    properdin s.
    reticuloendothelial s.
     (RES)
    staging s.
    two phase liquid culture s.

sys·te·moid

TA
   tubular adenoma

TAC
   total abdominal colectomy

Tac·a·ryl

TACE

Tac pep·tide

TAD
   6-thioguanine, cytarabine, and daunorubicin

Tag·a·met

talc

TAM
   tamoxifen

Tam
   tamoxifen

Ta·mof·en

ta·mox·i·fen cit·rate

tar·get·ing
   intracellular t.

TAR (thrombocytopenia–absent radius) syn·drome

tar·tra·zine

TATA

TATA fac·tor

tau·ro·cho·le·mia

tax·ol

TBI
   total body irradiation

TC-1 (stromal) cell line

Tc
   technetium

T-Cyp·i·o·nate

TDT
   tumor doubling time

TdT
   terminal deoxynucleotidyl transferase

Teb·a·mide

tece·leu·kin

Techne·Coll

Techne·Scan MAA

Techne·Scan PYP

tech·ne·ti·um
   t. Tc 99m
   t. Tc 99m albumin aggregated
   t. Tc 99m antimony trisulfide colloid
   t. Tc 99m gluceptate
   t. Tc 99m methylene diphosphonate
   t. Tc 99m pyrophosphate
   t. Tc 99m sulfur colloid

tech·nique
   Borchgrevink t.
   combined abdominal transsacral resection t.
   dilution-filtration t.
   Enzyme-Multiplied Immunoassay T.
   fluorescent antibody t.
   immunoperoxidase t.
   Ivy t.
   Laurell t.
   no-touch t.
   Oakley-Fulthorpe t.
   Ouchterlony t.
   Oudin t.
   peroxidase-antiperoxidase (PAP) t.
   sandwich t.
   split course t.

Tef·lon
   T. catheter

teg·a·fur

Teg·a·mide

Tega-Span

Teich·mann
   T's crystals

tek·no·cyte

tel·an·gi·ec·ta·sia
   ataxia-t.

tele·leu·kin

tele·ther·a·py

Tem·a·ril

Tem·po

Tenck·hoff
   T. catheter

ten·i·po·side

Ten-K

teno·syn·o·vi·tis
   nodular t.

ter·a·to·blas·to·ma

ter·a·to·car·ci·no·gen·e·sis

ter·a·to·car·ci·no·ma

ter·a·to·gen

ter·a·to·gen·e·sis

ter·a·to·ge·net·ic

ter·a·to·gen·ic

ter·a·to·ge·ni·ci·ty

te·ra·to·ma *pl.* te·ra·to·mas,
   te·ra·to·ma·ta
      benign t.
      benign immature t.
      benign mature t.
      immature t.
      malignant t.
      sacrococcygeal t.

te·ra·to·ma *(continued)*
      sacrococcygeal dermoid t.

ter·a·to·ma·ta

ter·a·to·ma·tous

ter·fen·a·dine

Tes·lac

test
      acid elution t.
      acidified serum t.
      alkali denaturation t.
      Ames t.
      antiglobulin t. (AGT)
      antiglobulin consumption
         t.
      Apt t.
      autohemolysis t.
      bentonite flocculation t.
      chemiluminescence t.
      coagulation t.
      complement fixation t.
      conglutinating comple-
         ment absorption t.
         (CCAT)
      contact t.
      Coombs' t.
      cyanide-ascorbate t.
      deoxyuridine suppression
         t.
      dexamethasone suppres-
         sion t.
      Donath-Landsteiner t.
      Duke's t.
      erythrocyte protoporphyrin
         (EP) t.
      euglobin clot lysis time t.
      euglobulin lysis t.
      Farr t.
      fecal occult blood t.
      flocculation t.
      Foshay's t.
      Francis' t.
      gel diffusion t.
      Gordon's biological t.
      Ham t.
      hapten inhibition t.

test *(continued)*
- hemadsorption t.
- hemagglutination inhibition t. (HI, HAI)
- hemoglobin t.
- histamine t.
- histamine flare t.
- Hoppe-Seyler t.
- Howell's t.
- immobilizaton t.
- indophenol t.
- intracutaneous t.
- intradermal t.
- Kelling's t.
- Kleihauer-Betke t.
- Kobert's t.
- Kveim t.
- leishmanin t.
- lepromin t.
- limulus t.
- lipase t.
- lupus band t.
- lymphocyte proliferation t.
- mallein t.
- microprecipitation t.
- MIF t.
- migration inhibitory factor (MIF) t.
- Mitsuda t.
- Moloney t.
- Montenegro t.
- multiple-puncture t.
- mumps skin t.
- NBT t.
- neutralization t.
- Nickerson-Kveim t.
- nitroblue tetrazolium (NBT) t.
- Oakley-Fulthorpe t.
- occult blood t.
- one-stage prothrombin time t.
- Ouchterlony t.
- Oudin t.
- partial thromboplastin time t.
- passive cutaneous anaphylaxis t.

test *(continued)*
- passive protection t.
- passive transfer t.
- patch t's
- PCA t.
- perimetry t.
- Pirquet t.
- platelet retention t.
- porphobilinogen t.
- Prausnitz-Küstner (P-K) t.
- precipitin t.
- protection t.
- prothrombin t.
- prothrombin consumption t.
- prothrombin-proconvertin t.
- pulmonary function t's
- Quick's t.
- radioallergosorbent t. (RAST)
- radioimmunosorbent t. (RIST)
- Ramon flocculation t.
- Rebuck t.
- Rose-Waaler t.
- Salomon's t.
- Sanford's t.
- scarification t.
- Schalfijew's t.
- Schultze's indophenol oxydase t.
- scratch t.
- serologic t.
- serologic t. for syphilis (STS)
- serum neutralization t.
- sheep cell agglutination t.
- Sia t.
- sickling t.
- skin t.
- skin window t.
- smear t.
- Stypven time t.
- sucrose lysis t.
- syphilis t.
- thromboplastin generation t.

test *(continued)*
    TPI t.
    TRAP t.
    Treponema pallidum complement fixation t's
    Treponema pallidum immobilization (TPI) t.
    two-stage prothrombin t.
    unheated serum reagin (USR) t.
    USR t.
    vanillymandelic acid spot t.
    VDRL (Venereal Disease Research Laboratory) t.
    von Pirquet t.
    Waaler-Rose t.
    Watson-Schwartz t.
    Wolff-Junghans t.

Tes·ta-C

Tes·ta·mone 100

Tes·ta·qua

Tes·tex

tes·tic·u·lar

tes·tic·u·lo·ma
    t. ovarii

test·ing
    tangent screen t.

tes·tis *pl.* tes·tes
    pulpy t.

Tes·to·ject-50

Tes·to·ject-LA

tes·to·lac·tone

Tes·tone-L.A.

tes·tos·te·rone
    t. propionate

Test·red

Tes·trin-P.A.

Te·su·loid

tet·ra·cy·cline

tet·ra·pla·tin

TG
    thioguanine

Tg
    thioguanine

6-TG
    6-thioguanine

6-Tg
    6-thioguanine

TGF-β
    transforming growth factor β

TGF-β₁
    transforming growth factor β₁

tha·las·sa·ne·mia

thal·as·se·mia
    α-t.
    β-t.
    δ-t.
    δβ-t.
    hemoglobin C–t.
    hemoglobin E–t.
    hemoglobin S–t.
    t. intermedia
    t. major
    t. minor
    sickle cell–t.

tha·las·so·po·sia

thal·li·um

the·co·ma
    luteinized t.

Thee·lin Aq·ue·ous

the·o·ry
    Cohnheim's t.
    dualistic t.
    monophyletic t.
    polyphyletic t.
    Ribbert's t.
    single hit t.

the·o·ry *(continued)*
    three-step t. of invasion
    trialistic t.
    unitarian t.

ther·a·py
    adjuvant t.
    AML consolidation t.
    anticoagulant t.
    L-asparaginase t.
    biologic t.
    biological response modi-
        fier t.
    blood component t.
    boron neutron capture t.
    chelation t.
    chemohormonal t.
    chemoradiation t.
    combined modality t.
    contact radiation t.
    diet t.
    dietary t.
    endocrine t.
    gene t.
    gene replacement t.
    hematoporphyrin t.
    heparin t.
    hormonal t.
    hormone t.
    immunosuppressive t.
    implantation radiation t.
    instillational t.
    interlesional t.
    interstitial radiation t.
    intracavitary t.
    intrathecal t.
    laser t.
    local t.
    metabolic t.
    monoclonal antibody t.
    multimodality t.
    neoadjuvant t.
    palliative t.
    palliative laser t.
    palliative radiation t.
    particle beam radiation t.
    photodynamic t.
    photoradiation t.

ther·a·py *(continued)*
    proton-beam t.
    PUVA (psoralen–ultravi-
        olet A) t.
    radiation t.
    radioiodine t.
    reprogramming t.
    salvage t.
    sanctuary t.
    systemic t.
    transfusion t.
    ultrasound t.
    whole-abdomen radiation
        t.

ther·mo·che·mo·ther·a·py

ther·mo·ra·dio·ther·a·py

ther·mo·sen·si·tive

ther·mo·sen·si·tiv·i·ty

thi·a·mine

thi·a·zole

thi·emia

thio·gua·nine

6-thio·guan·ine

thi·ol
    t. modification

thio·phos·phate

thio·pu·rine

6-thio·pu·rine

thio·sul·fate

thio·tepa

thio·urea

This·sen
    Roche-Wainer-T. method-
        ology

Tho·ma
    T.-Zeiss counting cell
    T.-Zeiss counting chamber

Thom·son
  Rothmund-T. syndrome

tho·ra·cen·te·sis

tho·ra·cot·o·my

THP-1 (monocytic leukemia)
  cell line

throm·ba·phe·re·sis

throm·base

throm·bas·the·nia
  Glanzmann's t.

throm·bin

throm·bin·o·gen

throm·bo·ag·glu·ti·nin

throm·bo·as·the·nia

throm·bo·cla·sis

throm·bo·clas·tic

throm·bo·cy·ta·phe·re·sis

throm·bo·cyte

throm·bo·cy·the·mia
  essential t.
  hemorrhagic t.
  idiopathic t., primary

throm·bo·cyt·ic

throm·bo·cy·to·crit

throm·bo·cy·tol·y·sis

throm·bo·cy·to·path·ia

throm·bo·cy·to·path·ic

throm·bo·cy·top·a·thy
  constitutional t.

throm·bo·cy·to·pe·nia
  amegakaryocytic t.
  congenital hypoplastic t.
  drug-induced t.
  gold-induced t.
  heparin-induced t.
  immune t.
  neonatal alloimmune t.

throm·bo·cy·to·pe·nia
  (continued)
    neonatal amegakaryocytic
    t.
    paraneoplastic t.
    X-linked t.

throm·bo·cy·to·poi·e·sis

throm·bo·cy·to·poi·et·ic

throm·bo·cy·to·sis
  essential t.
  reactive t.

throm·bo·elas·to·gram

throm·bo·elas·to·graph

throm·bo·elas·tog·ra·phy

throm·bo·em·bol·ic

throm·bo·em·bo·lism
  tumor t.

throm·bo·gen·e·sis

throm·bo·gen·ic

β-throm·bo·glob·u·lin

throm·bo·he·mor·rha·gic

throm·bo·ki·nase

throm·bo·ki·ne·sis

throm·bo·ki·net·ics

throm·bol·o·gist

throm·bol·y·sis

throm·bo·lyt·ic

throm·bo·mod·u·lin

throm·bon

throm·bo·path·ia

throm·bop·a·thy

throm·bo·pe·nia

throm·bo·pe·ny

throm·bo·phle·bi·tis
  migratory t.
  paraneoplastic t.

throm·bo·plas·tic

throm·bo·plas·tid

throm·bo·plas·tin
    extrinsic t.
    intrinsic t.
    tissue t.

throm·bo·plas·tin·o·gen

throm·bo·poi·e·sis

throm·bo·poi·et·ic

throm·bo·poi·e·tin

throm·bo·sis
    deep venous t. (DVT)
    venous t.

throm·bo·spon·din

throm·bo·sthe·nin

throm·bo·test

throm·box·ane

throm·box·ane syn·thase

throm·bus *pl.* throm·bi
    blood plate t.
    blood platelet t.
    coral t.
    fibrin t.
    hyaline t.
    plate t.
    platelet t.
    tumor t.

thrust
    proliferative t.

thy·mec·to·my

thy·mi·dine
    t. kinase
    t. monophosphate

thy·mi·dyl·ate syn·the·tase

thy·mi·tis

thy·mo·cyte
    cortical t.
    medullary t.

thy·mo·ma

thy·mo·me·tas·ta·sis

thy·mu·lin

thy·mus

thy·mus-de·pen·dent

thy·mus-in·de·pen·dent

thy·ro·glob·u·lin

thy·roid

thy·roid·ec·to·my

thy·roid·itis
    Hashimoto's t.

Thy·ro·lar

thy·rot·ro·pin

Thy·tro·par
    T.-Linberg operation

ti·azo·fur·in

Ti·con

Ti·gan

Ti·ject-20

Ti·khor

TIL
    tumor-infiltrating lympho-
        cyte

time
    activated partial thrombo-
        plastin t. (APTT, aPTT,
        PTT)
    ancrod t.
    bleeding t.
    bleeding t., secondary
    clot retraction t.
    clotting t.
    coagulation t.
    one-stage prothrombin t.
    partial thromboplastin t.
        (PTT)
    plasma clotting t.
    plasma recalcification t.

time *(continued)*
    t. to progression
    prothrombin t.
    recalcification t.
    reptilase t.
    Russell viper venom t.
    sedimentation t.
    thrombin t. (TT)
    tumor doubling t.
    t. without symptoms or
      toxicity (TWiST)

tis·sue
    bronchial-associated lym-
      phoid t. (BALT)
    connective t.
    extranodal t.
    gut-associated lymphatic t.
      (GALT)
    hematopoietic t.
    heterotopic t.
    lymphoid t.
    nodal t.

Tis·sue-Trol

ti·ter

Tit·ra·lac Plus

ti·trant

ti·trate

ti·tra·tion
    colorimetric t.
    complexometric t.
    coulometric t.
    potentiometric t.

tit·ri·met·ric

tit·rim·e·try

TLI
    total lymphoid irradiation

TN eryth·ro·cyte

TNF
    tumor necrosis factor

TNF-α
    tumor necrosis factor α

TNF-β
    tumor necrosis factor β

TNFR
    tumor necrosis factor re-
      ceptor

TNI
    total nodal irradiation

to·bac·co

to·coph·er·so·lan

Toi·son
    T's fluid
    T's solution

tol·bu·ta·mide

tol·er·ance
    high-dose t.
    high-zone t.
    immune t.
    immunologic t.
    low-dose t.
    low-zone t.
    self t.
    split t.

tol·er·ant

tol·er·a·tion

tol·ero·gen

tol·ero·gen·e·sis

tol·er·o·gen·ic

to·lo·ni·um chlo·ride

tol·u·i·dine
    t. blue O

to·mog·ra·phy
    bolus dynamic computed t.
    computed t.
    high-resolution computed
      t.
    positron emission t. (PET)
    single photon emission
      computed t. (SPECT)

topho·li·po·ma

topo·isom·er·ase
   t. II

Tor·res
   T. syndrome

tour·ni·quet
   scalp t.

tox·emia

tox·emic

tox·i·ce·mia

tox·ic·i·ty
   antibody-dependent cell-
      mediated t.
   bone marrow t.
   cardiac t.
   dose-limiting t.
   gonadal t.
   hematologic t.
   late t.
   renal t.
   time without symptoms of
      t. (TWiST)

tox·i·co·he·mia

TPA
   tissue plasminogen activa-
      tor

tPA
   tissue plasminogen activa-
      tor

t-PA
   tissue plasminogen activa-
      tor
   tissue-type plasminogen
      activator

TPC
   total proctocolectomy

T-10 pro·to·col

T-12 pro·to·col

tract
   aerodigestive t.
   biliary t.
   gastrointestinal t.

tract *(continued)*
   genitourinary t.
   urogenital t.

trait
   α-thalassemia t.
   β-thalassemia t.
   Fitzgerald t.
   Flaujeac t.
   Fletcher t.
   Hageman t.
   sickle cell t.
   Williams t.

TRAMPCOL
   6-thioguanine, daunorubi-
      cin, cytarabine, metho-
      trexate, prednisone, cy-
      clophosphamide,
      vincristine, and L-aspara-
      ginase

tran·ex·am·ic acid

trans-ac·ti·va·tion

tran·scrip·tion
   t. translation

trans·duc·tion
   signal t.

trans·fec·tion
   DNA t.

trans·fer
   adoptive t.

trans·fer·rin

trans·for·ma·tion
   blast t.
   blastic t.
   lymphocyte t.
   malignant t.
   neoplastic cell t.
   prolymphocytoid t.

trans·fu·sion
   autologous t.
   blood t.
   direct t.
   exchange t.

trans·fu·sion *(continued)*
    exsanguination t.
    granulocyte t.
    immediate t.
    indirect t.
    mediate t.
    plasma t.
    platelet t.
    t. reaction
    replacement t.
    substitution t.

trans·glu·tam·in·ase
    plasma t.

trans·la·tion
    nick t.
    transcription t.

trans·lo·ca·tion
    6;9 t.
    8;21 t.
    15;17 t.
    chromosomal t.
    reciprocal t.

trans·mi·gra·tion

trans·mis·sion
    transfusion-associated disease t.

trans·plant
    autologous bone marrow t.
    t. rejection

trans·plan·ta·tion
    allogeneic t.
    allogeneic bone marrow t.
    autologous t.
    autologous bone marrow t.
    bone marrow t.
    peripheral blood cell t.
    peripheral blood stem cell t.
    peripheral stem cell t.
    syngeneic t.
    syngeneic bone marrow t.
    syngenesioplastic t.
    xenogeneic bone marrow t.

trans·rec·tal

trans-ret·i·no·ic acid

trans·sa·cral

Tra·ve·nol In·fu·sor pump

treat·ment
    Beard's t.
    boost t.
    breast-conserving t.
    continuous t.
    fractionated t.
    multimodality t.
    PUVA (psoralen–ultraviolet A) t.
    radiation t.
    single-dose t.
    split-course t.
    unorthodox cancer t.
    Whipple's t.

Tré·lat
    Leser-T. sign

trend
    survival t.

treo·sul·fan

tres·to·lone ac·e·tate

tret·amine

Treves
    Stewart-T. syndrome

tri·al
    crossover t.

tri·al·ism

tri·am·cin·o·lone

tri·am·ter·ene
    t. and hydrochlorothiazide

tri·a·zene

tri·az·in·ate

Tri-B3

Tri·ban

Tri·benz·a·gan

trich·i·lem·mo·ma

tri·chlo·ro·ace·tic acid

tricho·ba·sal·i·o·ma hy·a·lin·i·cum

tricho·epi·the·li·o·ma
   t. papillosum multiplex

tri·cyc·lic nu·cleo·side phos·phate

tri·der·mo·ma

tri·eth·yl·ene·thio·phos·pho·ra·mide

tri·flu·pro·ma·zine

tri·glyc·er·ide

Tri-K

tri·ka·tes

Tri·la·fon Con·cen·trate

tri·lo·stane

Tri·ma·zide

tri·mep·ra·zine

tri·meth·o·ben·za·mide

tri·meth·yl·col·chi·cin·ic acid

tri·me·trex·ate
   t. glucuronate

tri·ni·tro·ben·zene

tri·ni·tro·ben·zene sul·phon·ic acid

tri·ni·tro·phen·yl

tri·pe·len·na·mine

tri·pro·li·dine

trip·to·rel·in pam·o·ate

tri·sac·cha·ride
   t's A and B

tris(2,3-di·bro·mo·pro·pyl) phos·phate

tri·so·my
   t. 8

Triz·ma

Troi·sier
   T's ganglion
   T's node
   T's sign

tropho·blas·to·ma

tro·po·my·o·sin

Trous·seau
   T's syndrome

tryp·to·phan

TSC
   technetium sulfur colloid

TSH
   thyroid-stimulating hormone

TSS
   transcription start site

TTF
   time to treatment failure

TTP
   thrombotic thrombocytopenic purpura
   time to tumor progression

tube
   Celestin's t.
   Souttar's t.

tu·ber·cle
   Farre's t's

tuft·sin

tu·mor
   Abrikosov's (Abrikossoff's) t.
   adenoid t.
   adenomatoid t.
   adipose t.
   adrenal t.
   aggressive t.
   alpha cell t.

tu·mor *(continued)*
    anaplastic t.
    anaplastic Wilms' t.
    aniline t.
    astrocytic t.
    benign t.
    beta cell t.
    bone t.
    borderline t.
    brain t.
    brainstem t.
    Brenner t.
    bronchial carcinoid t.
    Brooke's t.
    Brown-Pearce t.
    t. burden
    Burkitt's t.
    Buschke-Löwenstein t.
    carcinoid t.
    carcinoid t. of bronchus
    carotid body t.
    cartilaginous t.
    cellular t.
    central nervous system t.
    chest t.
    childhood t.
    choroid plexus t.
    CNS t.
    Codman's t.
    t. colli
    colloid t.
    connective-tissue t.
    craniopharyngeal duct t.
    cystic t.
    delta cell t.
    dermoid t.
    desmoid t.
    diarrheogenic t.
    diffuse t.
    dumb-bell t.
    eiloid t.
    embryonal t.
    embryonic gut–derived
       carcinoid t.
    embryoplastic t.
    encysted t.
    endocrine t.
    endodermal sinus t.

tu·mor *(continued)*
    endometrial sinus t.
    endometrioid t.
    epidermoid t.
    epidural spinal t.
    epithelial t.
    Ewing's t.
    exophytic t.
    t. extension
    extragonadal germ cell t.
    extramedullary spinal t.
    fatty t.
    fibrocellular t.
    fibroid t.
    fibroplastic t.
    focal t.
    fungating t.
    gastric carcinoid t.
    gelatinous t.
    germ-cell t.
    germinal t.
    giant cell t. of bone
    giant cell t. of tendon
       sheath
    glomus t.
    glomus body t.
    glomus jugulare t.
    granular cell t.
    granulosa t.
    granulosa cell t.
    granulosa–stromal cell t.
    granulosa–theca cell t.
    Grawitz's t's
    gross t.
    t. heating
    heterologous t.
    heterotypic t.
    high-grade t.
    histioid t.
    homoiotypic t.
    homologous t.
    Hortega cell t.
    Hürthle cell t.
    infiltrating t.
    t. infiltration
    innocent t.
    intracranial t.

tu·mor *(continued)*

intradural-extramedullary spinal t.
t. invasion
invasive t.
islet cell t.
ivory-like t.
Keasby t.
Krompecher's t.
Krukenberg's t.
lateral t.
localized t.
malignant t.
malignant mixed mesodermal t.
t. marker
melanotic neuroectodermal t.
Merkel cell t.
mesenchymal t.
midbrain t.
midline t.
migrated t.
migratory t.
mixed t.
mixed germ cell t.
mixed salivary gland t.
mucinous t.
mucoepidermoid t.
mucous t.
müllerian t.
multifocal t.
muscular t.
musculoskeletal t.
Nélaton's t.
nerve cell t.
neural crest t.
neuroectodermal t.
neuroepithelial t.
neurogenic t.
nonepithelial t.
noninvasive t.
nonseminomatous germ cell t.
ocular t.
organoid t.
oxyphil cell t.
Pancoast's t.

tu·mor *(continued)*

papillary t.
parotid gland t.
peripheral neuroectodermal t.
persistent t.
pineal region t.
placental site trophoblastic t.
plasma cell t.
polypoid t.
poorly differentiated large cell t.
posterior fossa t.
potato t.
premalignant fibroepithelial t.
primary t.
primitive neuroectodermal t.
pulmonary sulcus t.
Rathke's t.
Rathke's pouch t.
recurrent t.
residual t.
t. response
retinal anlage t.
rhabdoid Wilms' t.
sacrococcygeal t.
salivary gland t.
sand t.
sarcomatoid t.
Schmincke t.
Schwann-cell t.
Sertoli-Leydig cell t.
sex cord–stromal t.
sheath t.
skin t.
solid t.
spinal axis t.
spinal cord t.
t. spread
stereotaxic t.
subarachnoid t.
subcutaneous t.
superior sulcus t.
supratentorial t.
temporal bone t.

tu·mor *(continued)*
 teratoid t.
 transition t.
 tridermic t.
 true t.
 ulcerated t.
 undifferentiated small cell
  t.
 vaginal t.
 vascular t.
 villous t.
 Warthin's t.
 Wilms' t.
 yolk sac t.

tu·mor·af·fin

tu·mor·i·ci·dal

tu·mor·i·gen·e·sis

tu·mor·i·gen·ic

tu·mor·ous

tu·ni·ca
 t. albuginea

tu·ni·ca·my·cin

TUR
 transurethral resection

Tur·cot
 T. syndrome

Turn·bull
 T.-Cutait operation

turn·over
 erythrocyte iron t. (EIT)
 plasma iron t. (PIT)
 platelet t.
 red blood cell iron t. (RBC
  IT)

twin·ning
 MZ (monozygotic) t.

TWiST
 time without symptoms of
  toxicity

ty·lo·sis

type
 blood t's
 cell t.
 histological t.
 Hutchison t.

typ·ing
 t. of blood
 HLA t.
 platelet antigen t.
 primed lymphocyte t.
  (PLT)
 tissue t.

ty·ro·sine

ty·ro·sine ki·nase

ty·ro·sine phos·pha·tase

Tzanck
 T. preparation

U266 cell

U937 cell

Uce·phan

UGI (upper gastrointestinal)
se·ries

UIBC buf·fer re·agent

UICC
    International Union
        Against Cancer

UICC stag·ing (for melanoma)

ul·cer
    gastric u.
    Jacob's u.
    rodent u.

ul·cer·a·tion

ul·na *pl.* ul·nae

ul·tra·cen·trif·u·ga·tion

ul·tra·cen·tri·fuge

ul·tra·fil·ter

ul·tra·fil·trate

ul·tra·fil·tra·tion

ul·tra·mi·cro·pi·pet
    Doppler u.
    endocavitary u.
    intrarectal u.
    transrectal u.

ul·tra·struc·tur·al

Ul·tra-Tech·ne·Kow

ul·tra·vi·o·let

Ul·tra·zine-10

un·der·stag·ing

un·dif·fer·en·ti·at·ed

un·dif·fer·en·ti·a·tion

Un·dritz
    U. anomaly

Uni·gen

unit
    Bethesda u.
    burst-forming u.
    colony-forming u.
    colony forming u.-culture
        (CFU-C)
    colony forming u.-erythro-
        cyte (CFU-E)
    colony forming u.-granulo-
        cyte (CFU-G)
    colony forming u.-granulo-
        cyte-macrophage (CFU-
        GM)
    colony forming u.-macro-
        phage (CFU-M)
    colony forming u.-mega-
        karyocyte (CFU-meg)
    colony forming u.-stem cell
        (CFU-S)
    erythron burst-forming u.

u-PA
    urokinase-type plasmino-
        gen activator

UR
    unresectable

ure·thra

ure·thral

ure·threc·to·my

uric acid

uric·ac·i·de·mia

uri·case

uri·ce·mia

uro·bil·in·emia

uro·bi·lino·gen·emia

Uro·cit-K

uro·gas·trone

uro·gram

urog·ra·phy
    excretory u.
    intravenous u.

uro·ki·nase

Uro-KP-Neu·tral

Uro·mi·tex·an

uro·pod

uro·por·phy·rin·o·gen

uro·the·li·al

uro·the·li·um

uter·us *pl.* uteri

util·iza·tion
    red cell u. (RCU)

VA
villous adenoma

VAB-6
vinblastine, dactinomycin, bleomycin, cisplatin, cyclophosphamide

VABCD
vinblastine, doxorubicin, dacarbazine, lomustine, and bleomycin sulfate

VAC
vincristine, dactinomycin, and cyclophosphamide
vincristine, doxorubicin, and cyclophosphamide

vac·cine
bacille Calmette-Guérin (BCG) v.
BCG v.
melanoma v.
pneumococcal v.

VAD
vincristine, doxorubicin, and dexamethasone

va·gi·na *pl.* va·gi·nae

vag·i·nal

vag·i·nec·to·my

va·lence

Val·er·gen

Val·er·gen-10

Val·er·gen-20

VALG
Veterans Administration Lung Cancer Study Group

val·ue
buffer v.

val·ue *(continued)*
cryocrit v.
mean clinical v.
normal v's
reference v's

VAMP
vincristine, methotrexate, 6-mercaptopurine, and prednisone

va·nil·lyl·man·del·ic acid

Va·quez
Osler-V. disease

var·i·ant
CRM+ v.
CRM− v.
CRMᴿ v.
CRM-R v.
G.K. v.
Prower v.
Stuart v.

var·i·ce·al

var·ix *pl.* var·i·ces
esophageal v.

VASAG
Veterans Administration Surgical Adjuvant Cancer Chemotherapy Study Group

vas·cu·lar

vaso·pres·sin
arginine v. (AVP)

VATH
vinblastine, doxorubicin, thiotepa, and fluoxymesterone

VBAP
    vincristine, carmustine, doxorubicin, and prednisone

VBL
    vinblastine

Vbl
    vinblastine

VBM
    vinblastine, bleomycin sulfate, and methotrexate

VBP
    vinblastine, bleomycin and cisplatin

VCAM-1
    vascular cell adhesion molecule-1

VCR
    vincristine

Vcr
    vincristine

veg·e·ta·tion
    dendritic v.

vein
    portal v.

VeIP

Vel·ban

Vel·be

Vel·sar

ven·om
    Bothrops v.
    Calloselasma v.
    Cerastes cerastes v.
    Echis carinatus v.
    Russell's viper v.

ven·tric·u·lar

Ve·Pe·sid

ver·ap·a·mil

Ver·cyte

ver·do·he·min

ver·do·he·mo·chro·mo·gen

ver·do·he·mo·glo·bin

verge
    anal v.

Ver·o·cay
    V. bodies

vero·cy·to·tox·in

Ves·prin

Vet·er·ans Ad·min·is·tra·tion Lung Can·cer Stu·dy Group

V-Gan

V_H re·gion

vi·cine

view
    craniocaudal v.
    lateral v.
    oblique v.

vif gene

VIIa

VIIa re·com·bi·nant

VII Padua I

VII Ve·ro·na

VIIIc
    coagulant factor VIII

VIIIcag
    factor VIII coagulant antigen

VIIIrcf

VIIIvwf

vil·lo·ma

vil·lous

vin·blas·tine sul·fate

Vin·ca

Vin·ca·sar

Vin·ca·sar PFS

Vin·crex

vin·cris·tine sul·fate

vin·de·sine

vi·nyl
v. bromide
v. chloride

VIP
vasoactive intestinal poly-
peptide

vi·po·ma

Vir·chow
V's crystals
V's gland
V's law
V's node

vir·il·iza·tion

Vir·i·lon

vi·rus
Abelson leukemia v.
Abelson murine leukemia
v.
bovine leukemia v.
DNA tumor v.
Epstein-Barr v.
Esh sarcoma v.
Friend v.
Fujinami sarcoma v.
hepatitis B v. (HBV)
human immunodeficiency
v. (HIV)
tumor v.

vis·cos·i·ty
blood v.

Vis·ta·ject

Vis·ta·ject-25

Vis·ta·ject-50

Vis·ta·ril

Vis·ta·zine 50

vi·ta·min
v. A
v. B
v. B_2
v. B_6
v. B_{12}
v. C
v. D
v. deficiency
v. E
v. K
multiple v's

vit·ro·nec·tin

VLA
very late activation

VLA an·ti·gen

VLB,P
vinblastine and cisplatin

V_L re·gion

VM-26

VM-26PP

VMCP
vincristine, melphalan, cyclophosphamide, and
prednisone

vol·ume
blood v.
mean corpuscular v.
packed-cell v. (PCV)
v. of packed red cells
(VPRC)
plasma v.
red cell v.

vol·u·met·ric

von Clauss
v.C. method

von Hip·pel
v.H.-Lindau syndrome

von Wil·le·brand
asialo-v.W. factor
Minot-v.W. syndrome

von Wil·le·brand *(continued)*
  pseudo-v.W. disease
  v.W's factor

Von·trol

VP
  vindesine, cisplatin

VP-16
  etoposide

Vp-16
  etoposide

vul·va

vul·var

vul·vec·to·my

Vu·mon

vWD
  von Willebrand disease

vWF
  von Willebrand's factor

vWf
  von Willebrand's factor

vWF mul·ti·mer

Wain·er
    Roche-W.-Thissen methodology

Wal·den·ström
    hyperglobulinemic purpura of W.

Wal·dey·er
    W. factor
    W's ring

wall
    chest w.

Wall·hau·er
    W. and Whitehead's method

WAR
    whole abdominal radiotherapy

wart
    soot w.

War·thin
    W's tumor

Wash·ing·ton factor

Wat·son
    W.-Schwartz test

wave
    radiofrequency w.

WBRT
    whole-brain radiotherapy

WCSG
    Western Cancer Study Group

WDHA
    watery diarrhea with hypokalemic alkalosis

Wechs·berg
    Neisser-W. phenomenon

Wei·bel
    W.-Palade body

Weide·mann
    Beckwith-W. syndrome

Wei·gert
    W's iron hematoxylin solution

weight
    body w.

Weir
    Maunsell-W. operation

Weiss
    Haber-W. reaction

Well·co·vo·rin

Well·fe·ron

Wer·mer
    W's syndrome

Wer·ner
    W's syndrome
    W.-Schultz disease

Wes·ter·gren
    W. method
    W. sedimentation rate

Wes·tern blot

Wes·tern blot analysis

West·ern Can·cer Stu·dy Group

Whip·ple
    W. procedure
    W's treatment

White·head
    Wallhauser and W's method

Whit·more
    W. staging (for prostate cancer)

WHO (World Health
  Organization) clas·si·fi·ca·
  tion (of colorectal cancer)

WHO (World Health
  Organization) clas·si·fi·ca·
  tion (for central nervous
  system cancer)

Wi·dal
  Hayem-W. syndrome

Wil·le·brand
  W's syndrome

Wil·liams
  Fitzgerald-W.-Flaujeac
    factor
  W. factor
  W. trait

Wilms
  aniridia–W. tumor associ-
    ation
  W. tumor

Win·trobe
  W. and Landsberg's
    method
  W. hematocrit
  W. method

Wis·kott
  W.-Aldrich syndrome

Wolff
  W.-Junghans test

Work·ing For·mu·la·tion
  Clas·si·fi·ca·tion (for non-
  Hodgkin's lymphoma)

WR-2721
  amifostine

Wright
  W.-Giemsa stain

Wu
  Folin and W's method

xan·them·a·tin

xan·tho·as·tro·cy·to·ma
    pleomorphic x.

xan·thop·sis

xan·tho·sar·co·ma

xeno·ge·ne·ic

xeno·graft

xe·non
    x. Xe 133

Xe·non Xe 133-V.S.S.

xeno·trans·plant

XRT
    external radiation therapy

Ya·ki·ma
   hemoglobin Y.

yel·low

yel·low
   butter y.

Yo·shi-864

zac·o·pride

Zan·ca
    Z's syndrome

Zan·o·sar

Zan·tac

Zap·pert
    Z's chamber

Zeiss
    Abbé-Z. apparatus
    Abbé-Z. counting cell
    Abbé-Z. counting chamber
    Thoma-Z. counting cell
    Thoma-Z. counting cham-
      ber

ze·ta·crit

Ze·ta·fuge

Zim·mer·mann
    Z's elementary particles

zinc
    z. sulfate

zin·o·stat·in

Zol·a·dex

Zol·lin·ger
    Z.-Ellison syndrome

zone
    chemoreceptor trigger z.
    transition z.

Zo·ran

Zo·vir·ax

Human Blood Group Systems and Red Cell Antigenic Determinants

ABO Blood Group System

Antigenic Determinants

A (Subgroups A_1, A_2, A_3, A_m, A_o, A_x, A_{int}, A_{end}, A_{finn}, A_{el}, A_{bantu})
B (Subgroups B_3, B_x, B_{el})

Phenotype	Genotype
A_1	A^1A^1
	A^1A^2
	A^1O
A_2	A^2A^2
	A^2O
B	BB
	BO
A_1B	A^1B
A_2B	A^2B
O	OO
O_h (Bombay phenotype)	hh

Auberger Blood Group System

Antigenic Determinant

Au^a

Bg Blood Group System

Antigenic Determinants

Bg^a	Ho
Bg^b	Ho-like
Bg^c	Ot
DBG	Sto

231

Cartwright Blood Group System

Antigenic Determinants

Yt^a
Yt^b

Colton Blood Group System

Antigenic Determinants

Co^a
Co^b

Cost-Sterling Blood Group System

Antigenic Determinants

Cs^a
Yk^a

Diego Blood Group System

Antigenic Determinants

Di^a
Di^b

Dombrock Blood Group System

Antigenic Determinants

Do^a
Do^b

Duffy Blood Group System

Antigenic Determinants

Fy^a (*or* Fy1)
Fy^b (*or* Fy2)
Fy$^{a\,b}$ (*or* Fy3)
Fy4
Fy5

Phenotype

Phenotype	Genotype
Fy^{a+b-}	Fy^aFy^a
Fy^{a+b+}	Fy^aFy^b
Fy^{a-b+}	Fy^bFy^b
Fy^{a-b-}	Fy^oFy^o (or $FyFy$)

Gerbich Blood Group System

Antigenic Determinants

Ge 1
Ge 2
Ge 3

H Blood Group System

Antigenic Determinant

H

Phenotype	*Genotype*
H	*HH*
	Hh
h	*hh*

Ii Blood Group System

Antigenic Determinants

I
I^T
I^D
I^F
i

Kell Blood Group System

Antigenic Determinants

K1 (*or* K)
K2 (*or* k)
K3 (*or* Kp^a)
K4 (*or* Kp^b)
K5 (*or* Ku)
K6 (*or* Js^a)
K7 (*or* Js^b)
K8 (*or* kw)
K9 (*or* KL)
K10 (*or* $U1^a$)

K11 (*or* Côté)
K12 (*or* Bøk)
K13 (*or* Sgro)
K14 (*or* San)
K15 (*or* Kx)
K16 (*or* K-like)
K17 (*or* Wk^a)
K18
K19
Kp^c

Phenotype	Genotype
K + k −	KK
K + k +	Kk
K − k +	kk
Kp^{a+b+}	Kp^aKp^a
Kp^{a+b-}	Kp^aKp^b
Kp^{a-b+}	Kp^bKp^b
Js^{a+b-}	Js^aJs^a
Js^{a+b+}	Js^aJs^b
Js^{a-b+}	Js^bJs^b

Kidd Blood Group System

Antigenic Determinants

Jk^a (*or* Jk1)
Jk^b (*or* Jk2)
Jk$^{a\,b}$ (*or* Jk3)

Phenotype	Genotype
Jk^{a+b-}	Jk^aJk^a
	Jk^aJk
Jk^{a-b+}	Jk^bJk^b
	Jk^bJk
Jk^{a+b+}	Jk^aJk^b
Jk^{a-b-}	$JkJk$

Lewis Blood Group System

Antigenic Determinants

Le^a (*or* Le1)
Le^b (*or* Le2)
Le^c (*or* Le5)
Le^d
Le^x (*or* L^{ab} *or* Le3)
Mag (*or* Le4)

Phenotype	Genotype
Le^{a+b-}	*Le, ABO, H, sese*
	Le, hh, Se or *sese*
Le^{a-b+}	*Le, ABO, H, Se*
Le^{a-b-}	*lele, H, ABO, Se*
	lele, H, ABO, sese
	lele, hh, Se or *sese*

Lutheran Blood Group System

Antigenic Determinants

Lu^a (*or* Lu1)
Lu^b (*or* Lu2)
Lu$^{a\,b}$ (*or* Lu3)
Lu4
Lu5
Lu6
Lu7
Lu8
Lu9
Lu10
Lu11
Lu12
Lu13
Lu14 (*or* Sw^a)

Phenotype	*Genotype*
Lu^{a+b-}	*Lu^{a}Lu^a*
	Lu^{a}Lu
Lu^{a+b+}	*Lu^{a}Lu^b*
Lu^{a-b+}	*Lu^{b}Lu^b*
	Lu^{b}Lu
Lu^{a-b-}	*LuLu*
	In (Lu)

MNSs Blood Group System

Antigenic Determinants

Cl^a	N
Far	N^A
He	N^a
Hill	N$_2$
Hu	Ny^a
M	Ri^a
M$_1$	S
M^A	S$_2$
M^c	S^B
M^e	s
M^g	Sj
M^k	St^a
M^r	Sul
M^v	Tm
M^z	U
Mi^a	U^B
Mt^a	Vr
Mur	Vw
	Z

Phenotype / *Genotype*

Phenotype	Genotype
MS	*MS/MS*
MSs	*MS/Ms*
Ms	*Ms/Ms*
MNS	*MS/NS*
MNSs	*MS/Ns*
	Ms/NS
MNs	*Ms/Ns*
NS	*NS/NS*
NSs	*NS/Ns*
Ns	*Ns/Ns*

P Blood Group System

Antigenic Determinants

P1
P2 (Tj^a)
P3 (P^k)

Phenotype

P$_1$	P$_2^k$
P$_2$	p
P$_1^k$	Luke

Rh Blood Group System

Antigenic Determinants

Rosenfield Nomenclature	*Fisher-Race Nomenclature*	*Wiener Nomenclature*
Rh1	D	Rh_0
Rh2	C	rh′
Rh3	E	rh″
Rh4	c	hr′
Rh5	e	hr″
Rh6	ce *or* f	hr
Rh7	Ce	rh_i
Rh8	C^w	rh^{w1}
Rh9	C^x	rh^x
Rh10	V *or* ce^S	hr^v
Rh11	E^w	rh^{w2}
Rh12	G	rh^G
Rh13		Rh^A
Rh14		Rh^B
Rh15		Rh^C
Rh16		Rh^D
Rh17		Hr_0
Rh18		Hr
Rh19		Hr^S
Rh20	VS *or* e^s	
Rh21	C^G	
Rh22	CE	
Rh23	D^w	
Rh24	E^T	
Rh25	L^W	
Rh26	c-like	
Rh27	cE	
Rh28		hr^H
Rh29		RH
Rh30	D^{cor} (*or* Go^a)	
Rh31		hr^B
Rh32		
Rh33		
Rh34		Hr^B
Rh35		
Rh36		
Rh37		
Rh38		
Rh39		
Rh40		
Rh41		
Rh42	Ce^s	

Rh Blood Group System *(continued)*

Phenotype *(Wiener and Fisher-Race systems*)*	Genotype *(Wiener and Fisher-Race systems*)*
rh (ce)	*rr (cde/cde)*
rh'rh (Cce)	*r'r (Cde/cde)*
rh'rh' (Ce)	*r'r' (Cde/Cde)*
rh"rh (cCe)	*r"r (cdE/cde)*
rh"rh" (cE)	*r"r" (cdE/cdE)*
rh'rh" (CcEe)	*r'r" (Cde/cdE)*
rh_yrh (CcEe)	*$r^y r$ (CdE/cde)*
rh_yrh' (CEe)	*$r^y r'$ (CdE/Cde)*
$rh_yrh"$ (CcE)	*$r^y r"$ (CdE/cdE)*
rh_yrh_y (CE)	*$r^y r^y$ (CdE/CdE)*
Rh_0 (cDe)	*$R^0 R^0$ (cDe/cDe)* *$R^0 r$ (cDe/cde)*
Rh_1rh (CcDe)	*$R^1 r$ (CDe/cde)* *$R^1 R^0$ (CDe/cDe)* *$R^0 r'$ (cDe/Cde)*
Rh_1Rh_1 (CDe)	*$R^1 R^1$ (CDe/CDe)* *$R^1 r'$ (CDe/Cde)*
Rh_2rh (cDEe)	*$R^2 r$ (cDE/cde)* *$R^2 R^0$ (cDE/cDe)* *$R^0 r"$ (cDe/cdE)*
Rh_2Rh_2 (cDE)	*$R^2 R^2$ (cDE/cDE)* *$R^2 r"$ (cDE/cdE)*
Rh_1Rh_2 (CcDEe)	*$R^1 R^2$ (CDe/cDE)* *$R^1 r"$ (CDe/cdE)* *$R^2 r'$ (cDE/Cde)*
Rh_zrh (CcDEe)	*$R^z r$ (CDE/cde)* *$R^z R^0$ (CDE/cDe)* *$R^0 r^y$ (cDe/CdE)*
Rh_zrh_1 (CDEe)	*$R^z R^1$ (CDE/CDe)* *$R^z r'$ (CDE/Cde)* *$R^1 r^y$ (CDe/CdE)*
Rh_zRh_2 (CcDE)	*$R^z R^2$ (CDE/cDE)* *$R^z r"$ (CDE/cdE)* *$R^2 r^y$ (cDE/CdE)*
Rh_zRh_z (CDE)	*$R^z R^z$ (CDE/CDE)* *$R^z R^y$ (CDE/CdE)*

---

*Fisher-Race system in parentheses.

Sciana Blood Group System

Antigenic Determinants

Sm (*or* Sc1)
Bu^a (*or* Sc2)

Stoltzfus Blood Group System

Antigenic Determinant

Sf^a

Vel Blood Group System

Antigenic Determinants

Vel 1
Vel 2

Wright Blood Group System

Antigenic Determinants

Wr^a
Wr^b

Xg Blood Group System

Antigenic Determinant

Xg^a

Antigenic Determinants That Depend on Gene Interactions

ABO/I	IH, IA, IB, iH
P/I	IP1, IP2 (*or* IT$_j^a$), I^{T}P1, iP1
Lewis/I	ILe^{bh}
Lewis/ABO	A$_1$Le^b (*or* Seidler)
P/ABO	Luke
Xor/Duffy	Fy5
Rh/L^w	Rh25 (*or* L^w)

Selected Antigenic Determinants Not Yet Associated With a Blood Group System

754
An^a
At^a
Be^a
Bec
Bi
Big Charles
Bpa
Bra
Bxa
By
Cad
Car
Chido (or Gursha)
Chr^a
Cip
Coates
Craig
Dahl
Donaviesky
Dp
Driver
Duch
E1
En^a
Evans
Evelyn
Fin
Fuerhart
Fuj
Gf^a
Gilbraith
Gn^a
Go^b
Good
Green
Gy^a
Hands
Hen
Heibel
Hill
Ht^a
Hy
Je^a
Jn^a

Jo^a
Job
Jr
Kam
Kelly
Ken
Knops (or Kn^a)
Kosis
Lan
Lev
Lw^a
McCall
McCoy (or McC^a)
Man
Mar
Mo^a
MZ443
Nij
Ola
Orr
Pea
Pt^a
Rd^a
Reid
Rogers (or Rg^a)
Savior
Sch
Sd^a
Simon
Skjelbred
Ters
Th^a
To^a
Todd
Tr^a
Ven
Vennera
Wb
Weeks
Wil
Winbourne
Wu
Yh^a
York (or Yk^a)
Za

HLA (Human Leukocyte Antigen) Specificities

HLA-A

HLA-A1
HLA-A2
HLA-A3
HLA-A9
HLA-A10
HLA-A11
HLA-Aw19
HLA-A23
HLA-A24
HLA-A25
HLA-A26

HLA-A28
HLA-A29
HLA-A30
HLA-A31
HLA-A32
HLA-Aw33
HLA-Aw34
HLA-Aw36
HLA-Aw43
HLA-Aw66
HLA-Aw68
HLA-Aw69

HLA-B

HLA-Bw4
HLA-B5
HLA-Bw6
HLA-B7
HLA-B8
HLA-B12
HLA-B13
HLA-B14
HLA-B15
HLA-B16
HLA-B17
HLA-B18
HLA-B21
HLA-Bw22
HLA-B27
HLA-B35
HLA-B37
HLA-B38
HLA-B39
HLA-B40
HLA-Bw41
HLA-Bw42
HLA-B44
HLA-B45
HLA-Bw46

HLA-Bw47
HLA-Bw48
HLA-B49
HLA-Bw50
HLA-B51
HLA-Bw52
HLA-Bw53
HLA-Bw54
HLA-Bw55
HLA-Bw56
HLA-Bw57
HLA-Bw58
HLA-Bw59
HLA-Bw60
HLA-Bw61
HLA-Bw62
HLA-Bw63
HLA-Bw64
HLA-Bw65
HLA-Bw67
HLA-Bw70
HLA-Bw71
HLA-Bw72
HLA-Bw73

HLA-C

HLA-Cw1	HLA-Cw5
HLA-Cw2	HLA-Cw6
HLA-Cw3	HLA-Cw7
HLA-Cw4	HLA-Cw8

HLA-D

HLA-Dw1	HLA-Dw6
HLA-Dw2	HLA-Dw7
HLA-Dw3	HLA-Dw8
HLA-Dw4	HLA-Dw9
HLA-Dw5	

HLA-DP

HLA-DPw1	HLA-Dpw4
HLA-DPw2	HLA-DPw5
HLA-DPw3	HLA-DPw6

HLA-DQ

HLA-DQw1
HLA-DQw2
HLA-DQw3

HLA-DR

HLA-DR1	HLA-DRw9
HLA-DR2	HLA-DRw10
HLA-DR3	HLA-DRw11
HLA-DR4	HLA-DRw12
HLA-DR5	HLA-DRw13
HLA-DRw6	HLA-DRw14
HLA-DR7	HLA-DRw52
HLA-DRw8	HLA-DRw53

APPENDIX 3
Reference Values in Hematology

From Conn, R.B.: Laboratory Values of Clinical Importance. *In* Rakel, R.E. (ed.): Conn's Current Therapy 1993. Philadelphia, W.B. Saunders Company, 1993.

Reference Values in Hematology

		Conventional Units	SI Units
Acid hemolysis test (Ham)		No hemolysis	No hemolysis
Alkaline phosphatase, leukocyte		Total score 14–100	Total score 14–100
Cell counts			
Erythrocytes			
Males		4.6–6.2 million/mm³	4.6–6.2 × 10¹²/L
Females		4.2–5.4 million/mm³	4.2–5.4 × 10¹²/L
Children (varies with age)		4.5–5.1 million/mm³	4.5–5.1 × 10¹²/L
Leukocytes			
Total		4500–11,000 mm³	4.5–11.0 × 10⁹/L
Differential	*Percentage*	*Absolute*	*Absolute*
Myelocytes	0	0/mm³	0/L
Band neutrophils	3–5	150–400/mm³	150–400 × 10⁶/L
Segmented neutrophils	54–62	3000–5800/mm³	3000–5800 × 10⁶/L
Lymphocytes	25–33	1500–3000/mm³	1500–3000 × 10⁶/L
Monocytes	3–7	300–500/mm³	300–500 × 10⁶/L
Eosinophils	1–3	50–250/mm³	50–250 × 10⁶/L
Basophils	0–0.75	15–50/mm³	15–50 × 10⁶/L
Platelets		150,000–350,000/mm³	150–350 × 10⁹/L
Reticulocytes		25,000–75,000/mm³	25–75 × 10⁹/L
		0.5–1.5% of erythrocytes	
Coagulation tests			
Bleeding time (template)		2.75–8.0 min	2.75–8.0 min
Coagulation time (glass tubes)		5–15 min	5–15 min
Factor VIII and other coagulation factors		50–150% of normal	0.5–1.5 of normal
Fibrin split products (Thrombo-Welco test)		<10 µg/mL	<10 mg/L
Fibrinogen		200–400 mg/dL	2.0–4.0 g/L
Partial thromboplastin time (PTT)		20–35 sec	20–35 s
Prothrombin time (PT)		12.0–14.0 sec	12.0–14.0 s

Coombs' test		
Direct	Negative	Negative
Indirect	Negative	Negative
Corpuscular values of erythrocytes		
Mean corpuscular hemoglobin (MCH)	26–34 pg	0.40–0.53 fmol
Mean corpuscular volume (MCV)	80–96 μm³	80–96 fL
Mean corpuscular hemoglobin concentration (MCHC)	32–36%	0.32–0.36
Haptoglobin	26–185 mg/dL	260–1850 mg/L
Hematocrit		
Males	40–54 mL/dL	0.40–0.54 volume fraction
Females	37–47 mL/dL	0.37–0.47 volume fraction
Newborns	49–54 mL/dL	0.49–0.54 volume fraction
Children (varies with age)	35–49 mL/dL	0.35–0.49 volume fraction
Hemoglobin		
Males	14.0–18.0 gm/dL	2.17–2.79 mmol/L
Females	12.0–16.0 gm/dL	1.86–2.48 mmol/L
Newborns	16.5–19.5 gm/dL	2.56–3.02 mmol/L
Children (varies with age)	11.2–16.5 gm/dL	1.74–2.56 mmol/L
Hemoglobin, fetal	<1.0% of total	<0.01 of total
Hemoglobin A_{1C}	3–5% of total	0.03–0.05 of total
Hemoglobin A_2	1.5–3.0% of total	0.015–0.03 of total
Hemoglobin, plasma	0–5.0 mg/dL	0–0.8 μmol/L
Methemoglobin	30–130 mg/dL	4.7–20 μmol/L
Sedimentation rate (ESR)		
Wintrobe: Males	0–5 mm/hr	0–5 mm/h
Females	0–15 mm/hr	0–15 mm/h
Westergren: Males	0–15 mm/hr	0–15 mm/h
Females	0–20 mm/hr	0–20 mm/h